MAYO CLINIC

GUIDE TO

FIBROMYALGIA

MAYO CLINIC

Medical Editors
Andy Abril, M.D.
Barbara K. Bruce, Ph.D., L.P.

Editorial Director
Paula M. Marlow Limbeck

Senior Editor
Karen R. Wallevand

Managing Editor
Stephanie K. Vaughan

Senior Product Manager
Christopher C. Frye

Art Director
Stewart (Jay) J. Koski

Illustration, Photography and Production
Kent Mc Daniel, James (Jim) D. Postier II,
Gunnar T. Soroos

Editorial Research Librarians
Abbie Y. Brown, Edward (Eddy) S. Morrow Jr.,
Erika A. Riggin, Katherine (Katie) J. Warner

Copy Editors
Miranda M. Attlesey, Alison K. Baker,
Nancy J. Jacoby, Julie M. Maas

Indexer
Steve Rath

Contributing Reviewers and Writers
Rachel A. Haring Bartony; Susan M. Bee, APRN,
CNS; Florentina Berianu, M.D.; Ronald R. Butend-
ieck Jr., M.D.; Kenneth T. Calamia, M.D.; Pablo R.
Castillo, M.D.; Patricia M. Collins; Kari A. Cornell;
Kevin C. Fleming, M.D.; Jessica M. Gehin, R.N.;
Barbara J. Knox; Heather L. LaBruna; Connie A.
Luedtke, R.N., RN-BC; Arya B. Mohabbat, M.D.;
Shehzad K. Niazi, M.D.; Jane E. Ryan; Thomas D.
Rizzo Jr., M.D.; Jeffrey D. Rome, M.D.; Christopher
D. Sletten, Ph.D., L.P.; Benjamin Wang, M.D.;
Laura X. Waxman

Published by Mayo Clinic Press

For bulk sales to employers, member groups
and health-related companies, contact
Mayo Clinic, 200 First St. SW, Rochester, MN
55905, call 800-430-9699, or send an email to
SpecialSalesMayoBooks@mayo.edu.

ISBN 978-1-893005-50-1 (hard cover)
ISBN 978-1-893005-49-5 (softcover)

Library of Congress Control Number: 2019933030

Printed in the United States of America

Cover design by Stewart (Jay) J. Koski

Contents

VII

Letter from the editors

Every day, we see patients who hurt, aren't sleeping well, are exhausted and have trouble concentrating. By the time they get to us, many of these people have been told that their symptoms are from stress or depression. Others have been told that they're wasting their doctors' time. Some have even been told that they're crazy.

All the while, these people are struggling. They just want their lives back. They don't know what's wrong with them or how to make it better.

This is the story of fibromyalgia.

In our decades of experience at Mayo Clinic, we've worked with thousands of patients just like this — people with real symptoms of a real disorder known as fibromyalgia. We've seen these individuals use the strategies in this book to return to productive, fulfilling lives. You can do this, too.

Fibromyalgia is one of the most misunderstood disorders in medicine today. With *Mayo Clinic Guide to Fibromyalgia*, you'll learn the facts about this disorder and the science behind treatments that can help you manage it.

This book also offers hope. Hope that fibromyalgia doesn't have to define who you are. Hope that fibromyalgia doesn't have to ruin your life. Hope that you can return to a satisfying life, even with fibromyalgia.

We've watched as the strategies in this book have transformed lives. With these tools and techniques, people with fibromyalgia are returning to the lives they enjoy. You can, too.

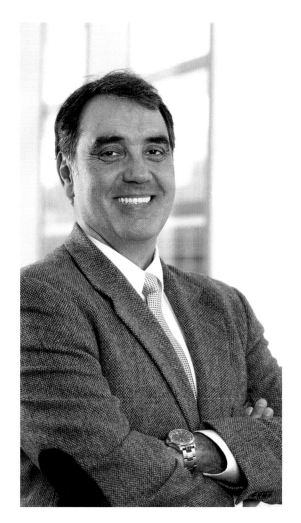

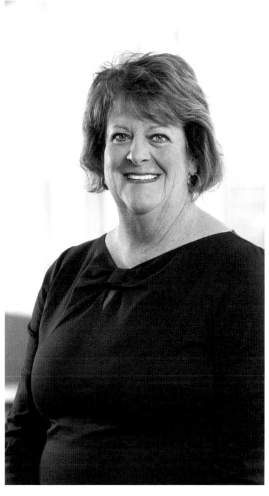

Andy Abril, M.D., is the chair of the Division of Rheumatology and co-medical director of the Fibromyalgia Treatment Program, a multidisciplinary program for treating fibromyalgia, at Mayo Clinic in Jacksonville, Fla. Dr. Abril is the program director of Mayo Clinic's Rheumatology Fellowship at the Florida campus, and an associate professor of medicine at the Mayo Clinic College of Medicine and Science. He is board certified in rheumatology.

Barbara K. Bruce, Ph.D., L.P., is the clinical director of the Fibromyalgia Treatment Program at Mayo Clinic in Jacksonville, Fla. She's also a pain psychologist in Mayo Clinic's Department of Psychiatry and Psychology and a professor of psychology at the Mayo Clinic College of Medicine and Science. Dr. Bruce is active in the American Pain Society and the International Association for the Study of Pain, as well as many other professional organizations dedicated to the study and treatment of pain.

How to use this book

Mayo Clinic Guide to Fibromyalgia is a comprehensive guide that provides answers and explanations about fibromyalgia. In this book, you'll learn what fibromyalgia is — and isn't — and how you can live a full, productive, enjoyable life with the condition. To help you easily find the information you're looking for, the book is divided into four sections.

Part 1: What is fibromyalgia?

This section covers all the basics about fibromyalgia. You'll get to know people who have fibromyalgia and learn about their experiences. If you're reading this book because you have fibromyalgia, you'll likely relate to the last chapter of this section, which outlines some of the condition's biggest challenges. Part 1 kick-starts your knowledge about fibromyalgia and sets the stage for managing it successfully.

Part 2: Treating fibromyalgia

In this section, you'll learn about fibromyalgia symptoms and how to manage them. In particular, you'll discover how cognitive behavioral therapy can help relieve your symptoms. You'll also learn about specific programs that teach cognitive behavioral therapies. Medications and integrative therapies also are addressed in this section.

Part 3: Managing symptoms

In this section, you'll use what you've learned about fibromyalgia and start developing techniques for managing your symp-

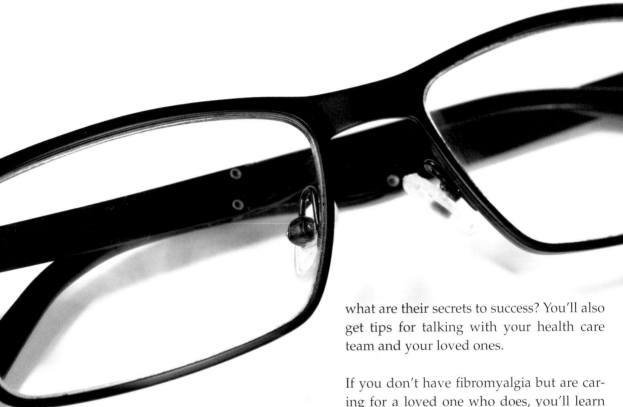

toms. You'll identify steps you can take, to successfully manage fibromyalgia.

Part 4: Living with fibromyalgia

To start this section, we'll revisit the people you read about at the beginning of the book. How are they managing fibromyalgia, and what are their secrets to success? You'll also get tips for talking with your health care team and your loved ones.

If you don't have fibromyalgia but are caring for a loved one who does, you'll learn how you can provide support. Part 4 closes with an action guide that brings together everything you've learned and puts it into a daily plan you can start using right away.

Finally, you'll find additional resources, including step-by-step exercise instructions, worksheets, and organizations you can contact for more information.

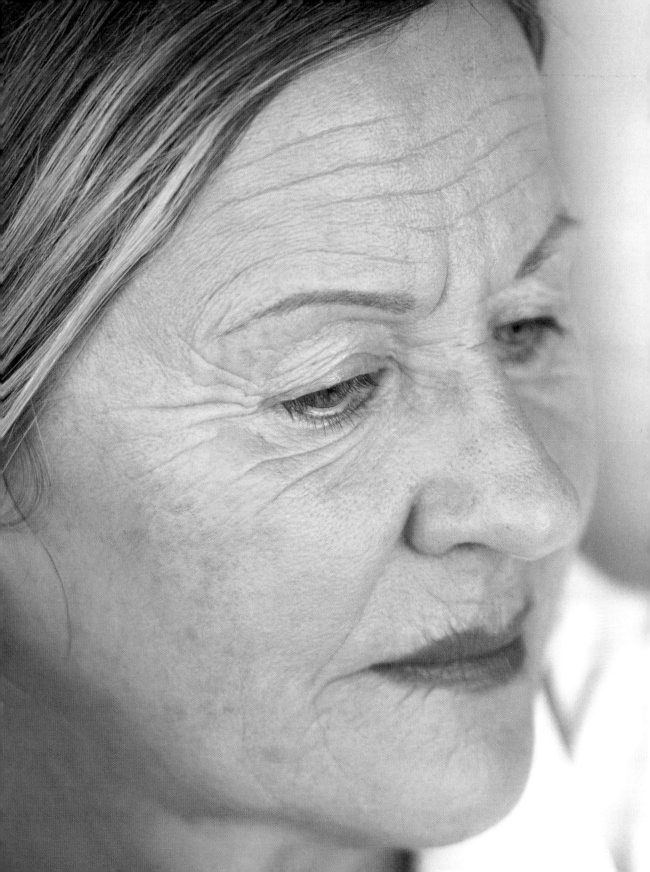

PART 1

What is fibromyalgia?

Your muscles ache. Your joints hurt. Your neck feels stiff. Your thinking often seems muddled. You're exhausted. You feel light-headed sometimes. You can't sleep — or, all you want to do is sleep more.

With fibromyalgia, you may feel all of this — and more — but have no idea why. To make things worse, maybe you've had every medical test imaginable, yet your doctor can't say what's causing your symptoms.

The key to remember in all of this is that the symptoms you're feeling are real. Fibromyalgia is a real condition. It's also a treatable condition. There are ways fibromyalgia can be managed, which you'll learn about in this book.

In Part 1, you'll get a better understanding of what fibromyalgia is and what it isn't. You'll get to know its signs and symptoms — and why it's so hard to diagnose. You'll also discover the many effects of this condition. Fibromyalgia can touch your life in more ways than you might imagine.

Getting to know more about fibromyalgia is the first step toward managing it and living your best life now. Let's get started.

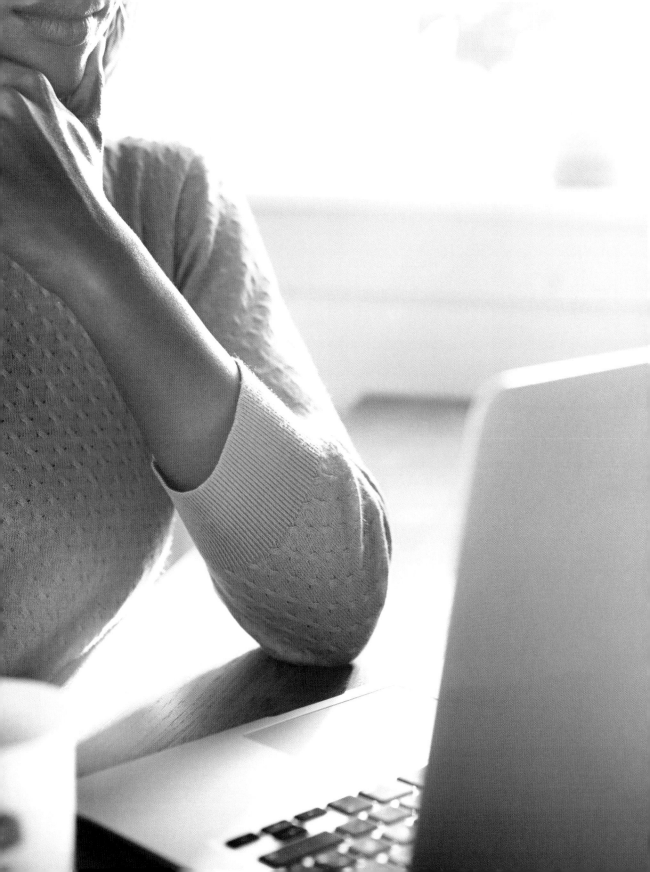

CHAPTER 1

A brief introduction

Fibromyalgia is often misunderstood. Some people believe it isn't real, or that its symptoms are signs of depression, stress or any other number of other conditions.

Mayo Clinic Guide to Fibromyalgia dispels common myths like these and outlines the facts about fibromyalgia. Fibromyalgia is, indeed, a real condition. It's a sensory disorder caused by a miscommunication between the nerves throughout your body and your brain. And it's treatable.

In the pages that follow, you'll learn what researchers have uncovered about fibromyalgia — what it is, what it isn't and what causes it. Better yet, by the time you get to the end of this book, you'll have a set of research-supported tools and strategies to manage your fibromyalgia symptoms so that you can return to the life you enjoy.

People who use the strategies in this book say that they help lessen the effect fibromyalgia has on their lives. They feel less pain and are less tired and depressed.

If you have fibromyalgia, you may wonder what steps you should take and how to begin your treatment plan. If you think you might have fibromyalgia but don't know for sure, you may not know where to turn. Or maybe you're reading this book because someone you care about has fibromyalgia, and you're not sure how to help. This book is for every one of you.

Page by page, this book offers guidance and hope that fibromyalgia doesn't have to rule your life. You can live well with this condition, and the pages that follow will teach you how. Let's start the journey by meeting two people with fibromyalgia.

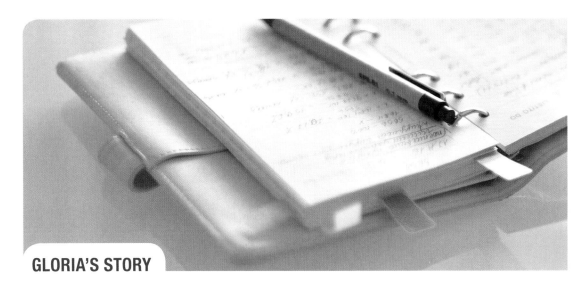

GLORIA'S STORY

'I hadn't even heard of fibromyalgia'

Gloria likely had been dealing with fibromyalgia for 20 years but didn't know it.

It isn't surprising that it took so long for Gloria to learn that she has fibromyalgia. When her symptoms first appeared, the term fibromyalgia was barely known.

Gloria's medical history is also anything but simple. She's had kidney, bladder and reproductive issues. At one point, she was in and out of the hospital for a month because of a viral illness.

Gloria has also faced her fair share of stress. Her son was born with a heart defect, her daughter with a chest deformity. And her husband's work took the family on several cross-country moves.

By 2001, Gloria was struggling. It became difficult for her just to get through each day.

She was having trouble sleeping. She was tired all the time, and she felt worse by the day. "I ached from my head to my toenails," Gloria said.

It seemed that any one — or any combination — of the life events Gloria was experiencing could be causing her symptoms. So Gloria met with doctors. After a thorough workup, she was told she had fibromyalgia.

At first, Gloria wasn't sure what to think. "I remember asking myself, *What will they call it next?*" A condition that had taken on many different names over the years (learn more starting on page 21), Gloria recalls, "I hadn't even heard of fibromyalgia."

Find out how Gloria learned to manage her fibromyalgia and how she's doing today later in this book (see page 192). You'll also hear from Gloria's husband and get his point of view on supporting someone with fibromyalgia on page 212.

"You ache, you hurt, your muscles ache, your joints hurt. Every nerve in my body just begins to pulsate under my skin. Sometimes it's like every nerve is on fire. I could be standing at the sink doing dishes, and I feel like someone stuck me with a needle [along] those points in your body that they test. Oftentimes, [I'll] get a sudden, stabbing pain in one of those areas for no reason at all."

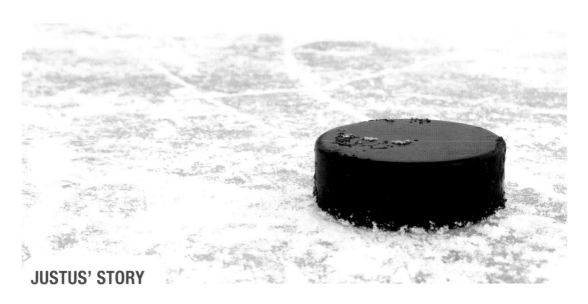

JUSTUS' STORY

'I just couldn't shake the pain'

At age 24, Justus may be the last person you'd think of when you picture someone with fibromyalgia. After all, the statistics are clear: More women than men experience fibromyalgia, and the condition often affects women who are middle-aged. But Justus isn't alone, and he's proof-positive that anyone of any age can have fibromyalgia.

Justus' journey with fibromyalgia likely started even before he was a teenager. At age 12, he was playing ice hockey and recalls asking his mom to rub his knees, ankles, calves and elbows. His aches and pains eventually led him to a chiropractor and a massage therapist. As Justus continued to grow, so did his participation in sports. He played football and baseball and boxed. He planned to play baseball in college. But at

"I JUST COULDN'T SHAKE THE EVERYDAY PAIN ... IT WAS HARD EVERY MORNING TO GET UP."

the same time, he always hurt. The pain came to a head when Justus turned 17.

"I ended up pulling my hip flexor off my hip and breaking my hip in the process. I spent my 17th birthday in the hospital," Justus says. This led him to stop playing baseball.

When Justus went to college, his pain followed him there. "I just couldn't shake the everyday pain, the waking up and feeling like I got hit by a cement truck," Justus says. "It was hard every morning to get up. My muscles ached and they hurt, and it didn't matter if I worked out the day before or if I stayed home all day. It was the same kind of pain."

Justus managed to earn his degree and chose to continue his schooling. But then he hit a wall.

"It was getting to be too much," Justus said. "Not only is the pain affecting me, but now it's starting to affect my mind and how I'm thinking about things and how I'm thinking about life. The everyday struggle of waking up and not knowing [what was wrong] would put me in a place where — not that I wanted to kill myself, but I was in a place

where I didn't necessarily want to wake up because I knew waking up would involve dealing with the pain again and not knowing [what was causing it]."

Questions started to swirl in his mind. *Do I want to keep doing this every single day? Who do I talk to? Is this just in my head? Am I making this up? Is this even really happening? I look like I'm healthy, but I don't feel like I'm healthy.*

Friends couldn't understand what he was going through, and that added to his misery, mentally and emotionally. Doctor after doctor had no answer to explain his symptoms. Justus felt alone and unsure of what to do.

With his parents by his side, Justus went from doctor to doctor and clinic to clinic in search of an answer that would explain his symptoms. Ultimately, Justus learned he had fibromyalgia. He was shocked and angry when he was told he had a condition that wasn't going to go away. He was 22 years old.

"I was so angry when I was diagnosed," Justus said. "Angry at God and angry at the situation and angry at anyone associated with [fibromyalgia] because they said I had this condition that they said is probably going to be for the rest of my life, and they say there's no cure for it. And so that made me angry."

Doctors told Justus about a three-week pain rehabilitation program that could help him, but he wasn't ready for it. *I can do this on my own,* Justus told himself. *I can figure this out.* He read everything he could get his hands on and found videos to watch, all with the hope that he would be able to figure out how to manage his symptoms on his own.

Eleven months later, Justus reached his breaking point. *I'm never going to be able to figure this out on my own,* he remembers thinking. That's when he signed up for and took part in the rehabilitation class. Through the program, Justus learned ways he could manage his symptoms without medication and improve his quality of life.

Learn what steps Justus took to manage his fibromyalgia and how he's doing today on page 194.

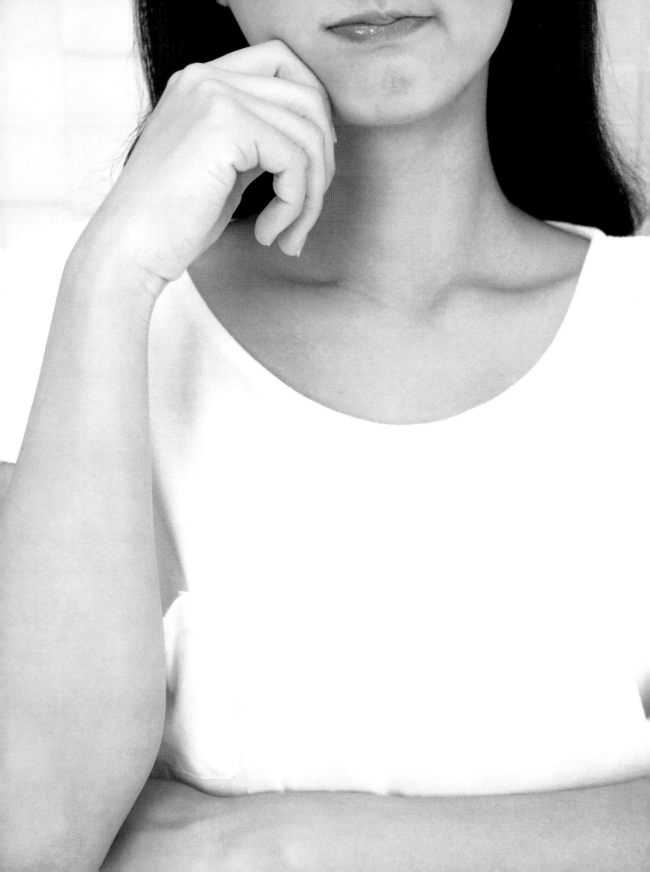

CHAPTER 2

Fibromyalgia's lengthy journey

Through the stories Gloria and Justus shared in the last chapter, you got an inside look at what living with fibromyalgia is like day to day. If you have fibromyalgia, you may be able to relate to their experiences, or at least parts of them. Their symptoms may have sounded familiar to you.

With all of this in mind, let's back up a step: What exactly is fibromyalgia?

In this chapter, you'll learn about the history of fibromyalgia and the twists and turns that this condition has taken over time, leading to what experts and researchers know about it today.

NEW CONDITION OR ANCIENT HISTORY?

As diseases go, fibromyalgia may seem like one of the newer kids on the block. But is it really? It's true that as far as *recorded* history is concerned, fibromyalgia goes back only 40 years or so — 1976, specifically. But a little more digging shows that it has roots that are hundreds, if not thousands, of years old.

Early origins

Fibromyalgia may date all the way back to biblical times, in particular, to the story of Job. Job said that "gnawing pains" that would "take no rest" led to restless nights. If you have fibromyalgia, you may be able to relate to what this feels like. Back then, chronic pain that didn't seem to have a cause and couldn't be treated was seen as punishment sent from beyond.

This idea of pain as punishment lasted until fourth century B.C. That's when Hippocrates, known as the Father of Medicine, came up with the theory that pain had a natural cause. He thought that the brain was sending fluid to the lower limbs, and this led to pain in the body. More fluid meant swelling and inflammation, which caused the pain.

When medical records came into the picture, so did descriptions of aches and pains now linked to fibromyalgia. In 1592, French physician Dr. Guillaume de Baillou came up with the word *rheumatism* to describe joint and muscle pain. Rheumatism describes pain, discomfort, soreness and stiffness that can affect how easily you move. The terms he used to describe muscle and joint aches are still used today.

Experts continued to study rheumatism into the 18th and early 19th centuries. They learned that it affected not just joints but also muscles and the body's soft tissues. They also found that fatigue and sleep problems were common, along with muscle pain and stiffness.

Tender points, trigger points and nodules — common terms used in describing fibromyalgia — came into the picture in the 19th century. To sum them up briefly, tender points are painful areas of tenderness. Trigger points are areas of the body that, when touched, cause pain in other parts of the body. And nodules are hardened areas of muscle that are painful to the touch.

All of these terms played a role in how the understanding of fibromyalgia has taken shape over the years. In fact, they've all helped lead to today's understanding of the condition: that fibromyalgia is caused by a glitch in the way the nervous system processes pain. You'll learn more about this in Chapter 4.

More recent developments

Until the late 19th century, doctors thought that the changes in the nervous system that led to fibromyalgia must have a physical cause. But toward the end of the century, this idea changed. That's when an American neurologist came up with the theory that the symptoms of fibromyalgia resulted from life's stresses.

The idea was that mental or emotional trauma, such as the death of a loved one, business or family troubles, and childbirth, were examples of situations that caused stress overload for some people. In turn, this overload of stress led to fibromyalgia.

Nearly a century later, this theory held true. Soldiers admitted to a British army hospital complained of widespread aches and pains that didn't seem to have a physical cause.

The soldiers all had two things in common: depression and stress. Similar cases were seen in U.S. military hospitals at the same time. Fifty years later, soldiers with Gulf War syndrome had the same symptoms.

This doesn't mean that fibromyalgia is all in a person's head. However, these experiences do suggest that physical and psychological trauma may be a cause of fibromyalgia.

In the early 20th century, the term *fibrositis* came into use. Doctors used this term to describe discomfort caused by swelling in the muscles. This term was used for the next seven decades. Widespread pain, tender points, fatigue and sleep problems were all symptoms of fibrositis. Today, all of these are known symptoms of fibromyalgia.

By the 1950s, fibrositis became a catch-all diagnosis for people who reported puzzling symptoms. In time, fibrositis was broken down into two types: generalized and localized. The generalized form of fibrositis would come to be known as fibromyalgia.

In the 1960s, the term *fibrositis* started to include other symptoms. In turn, a description that's fairly similar to what's used for fibromyalgia today was born. This led to a set of criteria, published in the early 1970s, that provided the first modern description of what was yet to be called fibromyalgia.

It was in 1976 that the term *fibromyalgia* finally emerged. Its roots lie in Latin and Greek: *fibra* for "fibrous tissue," *myos* for "muscles," and *algos* for "pain."

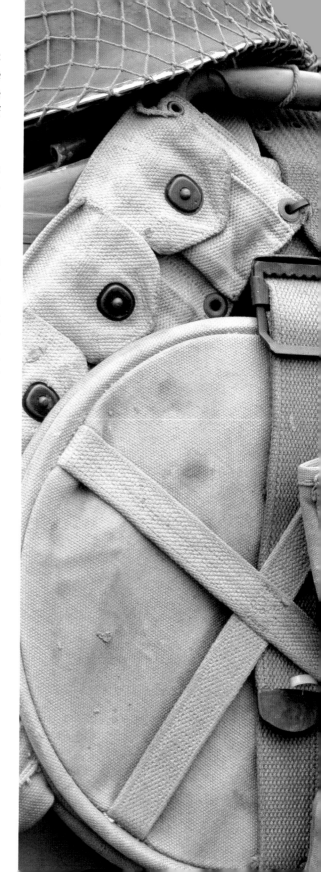

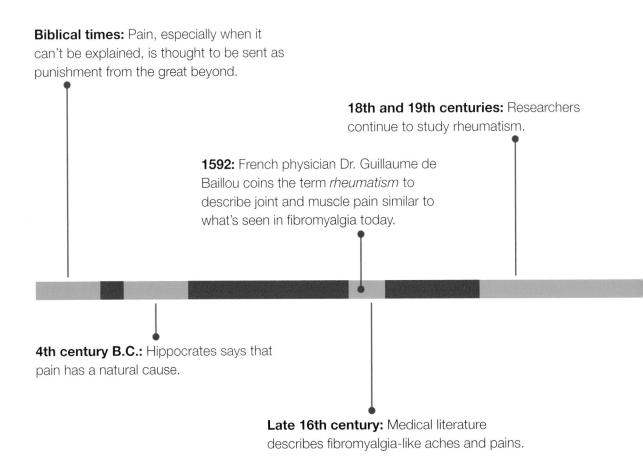

Biblical times: Pain, especially when it can't be explained, is thought to be sent as punishment from the great beyond.

18th and 19th centuries: Researchers continue to study rheumatism.

1592: French physician Dr. Guillaume de Baillou coins the term *rheumatism* to describe joint and muscle pain similar to what's seen in fibromyalgia today.

4th century B.C.: Hippocrates says that pain has a natural cause.

Late 16th century: Medical literature describes fibromyalgia-like aches and pains.

1824: Eventually seen as a symptom of fibromyalgia, painful areas of tenderness, called tender points, are discovered.

1976: The term *fibromyalgia* is first used.

1904: British neurologist Sir William Gowers introduced the term *fibrositis.* Widespread pain, tender points, fatigue and sleep problems are all symptoms of fibrositis.

Early 1970s: A set of criteria provided the first modern description of what would eventually be called fibromyalgia.

1950s: The term *fibrositis* became a catch-all diagnosis for people who reported puzzling symptoms.

1939-1940s: During and after World War II, soldiers admitted to a British army hospital complained of widespread aches and pains that didn't seem to have a physical cause. They all had two things in common: depression and stress. Similar cases were seen in U.S. military hospitals.

1869: American neurologist Dr. George Beard comes up with the term *neurasthenia*. It means nervous exhaustion and was used to describe symptoms that are now known to be common in fibromyalgia. Dr. Beard blamed the symptoms on life's stresses.

1960s: Fibrositis started to include other symptoms, leading to a description that's fairly similar to what's used for fibromyalgia today.

First a term, then a definition

With an accepted term in place, interest in the condition exploded. Many doctors, unfamiliar with how to recognize and diagnose it, wanted to learn more. It was time for an answer to everyone's burning question: What exactly is fibromyalgia?

Coming up with an agreed-upon list of symptoms for a fibromyalgia diagnosis would be a feat. Researchers from all over the globe had to weigh in, and there were a lot of differing opinions to sift through.

After years of discussion and debate, a group of organizations produced The 1990 American College of Rheumatology Criteria for the Classification of Fibromyalgia. With a list of agreed-upon symptoms in place, this virtually unknown condition moved closer to becoming a household word. Just a few years later, the advent of the internet offered a buffet of fibromyalgia information to anyone at any time.

With this sudden influx of information came new challenges. Doctors, patients, drug manufacturers and insurance companies all had questions. "Is there a medical test to prove someone has fibromyalgia?" "Is it a psychiatric disorder?" "When it comes to disability payments … how long and how much?" "What drugs are used to treat it?" "How many doctor visits does someone with fibromyalgia need every year?"

People needed help understanding this condition. To that end, experts got together to revise the 1990 criteria three different times (learn more in Chapter 5). As new discoveries shed new light on fibromyalgia, they'll no doubt be revisited again.

WHAT EXPERTS KNOW TODAY

Clearly, the understanding of fibromyalgia has evolved over time. Ancient Greeks thought that the pain started in the brain. Centuries later, experts focused on the muscles as the cause. Mental and emotional factors have been blamed, as well.

No matter what was considered the cause over the years, one thing has remained the same: Fibromyalgia is a pain disorder.

Today, a whole-person approach is becoming the standard of care. For example, when doctors diagnose fibromyalgia, they look far beyond just pain. They now know that other symptoms are at play, too. Doctors also realize now that each person's experience with the condition is different and that symptoms can wax and wane.

Why the new outlook? Improvements in brain imaging and pain testing have pulled back the veil on the cause of fibromyalgia. This has helped many doctors feel more confident about spotting fibromyalgia in the first place.

For example, newer imaging techniques used in research have helped doctors to see that fibromyalgia is linked to changes in the central nervous system.

A CONDITION WITH MANY NAMES

The term *fibromyalgia* has been in place since 1976. Before then, it went by quite a few different names. Each name offers a clue as to what researchers thought was the most likely cause of the condition. Swollen tissues, nerve problems and tense muscles were among the symptoms that played roles in the names fibromyalgia has gone by. You'll see that the suffix *-algia* is common. It's the Greek word for "pain."

Year	Term	Year	Term
1592	Rheumatism	1930	Allergic toxemia
1841	Neuralgia	1937	Psychogenic rheumatism
1843	Muscle calluses	1940	Idiopathic myalgia
1876	Chronic rheumatic myitis	1941	Rheumatic myalgia
1880	Neurasthenia	1950	Tension myalgia
1904	Fibrositis	1951	Allergic myalgia
1911	Nodular fibromyositis	1952	Myofascial pain syndrome
1919	Muscle gelling	1955	Myodysneuria
1921	Muscle hardening	1970	Generalized tendomyopathy
1927	Myofasciitis	1973	Interstitial myofibrositis
1929	Myofibrositis	1976	Fibromyalgia
1930	Neurofibrositis		

"WITH THE RIGHT BLEND OF STRATEGIES ... YOU CAN MANAGE THIS CONDITION."

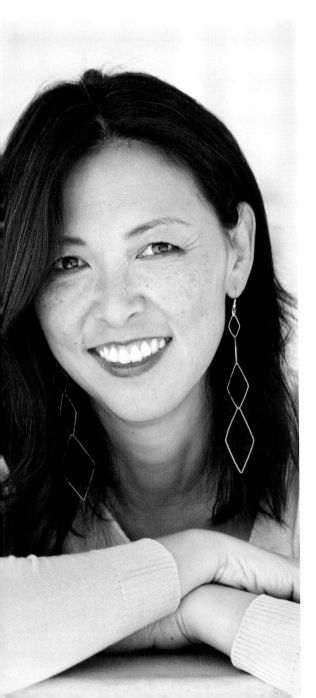

In particular, fibromyalgia is thought to be caused by a disorder called central sensitization (learn more about this on page 47).

While experts know a lot more about fibromyalgia today than they did centuries ago, research continues. In the next couple of chapters, you'll gain more insights based on what the latest evidence shows.

WHAT FIBROMYALGIA IS NOT

Now that you know a little bit about the history of fibromyalgia and how viewpoints have evolved over time, let's talk about what fibromyalgia is *not*. This will set the stage for Chapter 3, which dives into common myths and facts about the condition.

Fibromyalgia isn't deadly

If you don't know a lot about this condition but have been diagnosed with it, you may be afraid. Afraid of what it is and how it will change your life. Thousands of questions may be zipping through your brain. One question — "Will I die of this?" has a short, simple answer: no.

Unlike illnesses that can be terminal, such as cancer, fibromyalgia doesn't shut down your major organs or cause tumors to grow and spread throughout your body. It doesn't harm your joints, muscles or internal organs. It also doesn't make it more likely that you'll die an earlier death.

At the same time — and you likely already know this — fibromyalgia will change your life. But the changes aren't dire, and they're changes you can cope with. You'll learn how as you read this book. With the right blend of strategies and a supportive network of friends and family, you can manage this condition.

Fibromyalgia isn't a progressive disease

A disease that's progressive spreads or worsens over time. Take multiple sclerosis, for example. It often leads to nerve damage and causes someone to lose the use of muscles. This happens over time — that's what makes it progressive. Fibromyalgia doesn't damage your body over time, so it's not a progressive disease. However, the symptoms may worsen at times.

And although fibromyalgia isn't progressive, it can *feel* progressive. You may also feel as though you're losing ground over time. It may feel harder to get up the stairs this morning or walk to the mailbox today than it did yesterday. But fibromyalgia isn't what's causing these changes. Instead, your level of conditioning is the culprit.

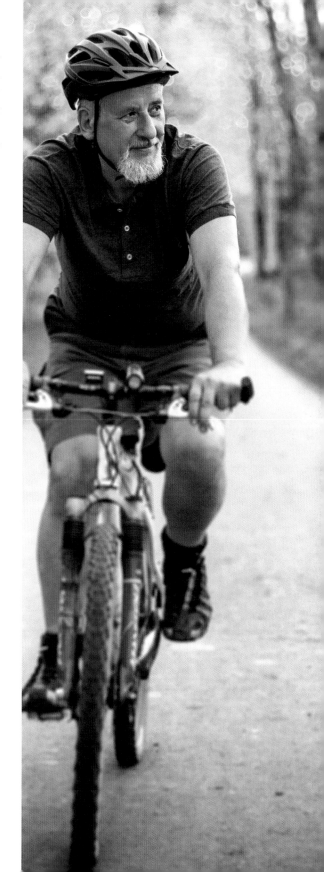

"IT'S IMPORTANT TO REMEMBER THAT THE SYMPTOMS YOU EXPERIENCE WITH FIBROMYALGIA ARE REAL."

Here's how it works. The pain and fatigue of fibromyalgia may lead you to do less over time. When you use your muscles less, you become weaker.

If pain and fatigue have you moving simply from bed to chair or from recliner to couch, you are doing less and less. This means you're becoming deconditioned. And as you become more and more deconditioned, daily tasks seem harder to do — or even impossible. When this happens, you may stop going upstairs or sweeping the porch altogether. When you stop doing the daily tasks of living, this is actually what makes you become deconditioned.

The good news is that you can completely regain all of the strength that you feel you have lost. You'll learn how in Chapter 13.

Fibromyalgia isn't a chronic infection, such as Lyme disease

If you've ever had a chronic infection, such as Lyme disease, you may see some similarities between the symptoms you had then and the symptoms you have with fibromyalgia. Fatigue, joint pain, muscle pain and stomach issues are among them.

While some symptoms of a chronic infection may mimic fibromyalgia, fibromyalgia itself isn't a chronic infection. However, a serious infection can trigger fibromyalgia (learn more on page 51).

Having fibromyalgia doesn't make you a hypochondriac

Perhaps you never used to worry about your health. But now, with fibromyalgia, maybe you've become concerned about the symptoms that this condition creates on a daily basis. You may wonder a number of things: *Am I having a heart attack? Do I have appendicitis? Do I need to go to the emergency room? Do I have a brain tumor? Did I somehow break my ankle?*

It's not uncommon for someone with fibromyalgia to visit doctor after doctor for some time before finally receiving a diagnosis. In fact, it can take several years to get a diagnosis. After completing a series of tests, all with normal results, your doctor may feel that your symptoms aren't real or blame them on depression or stress.

In the meantime, your family and friends may think you're a person who complains about symptoms that aren't real (hypochondriac).

It's important to remember that the symptoms you experience with fibromyalgia *are* real. The term *health anxiety* may better describe what you're feeling.

Before learning they have fibromyalgia, many people feel isolated and begin to question if what others are saying might be true. You may have asked yourself, *Am I losing my mind? Is it all in my head?* Even though more is known today than ever before about this condition, questions still remain, and fibromyalgia is still often underdiagnosed and undertreated.

Through it all, the bottom line to always remember is this: Your symptoms are real, and fibromyalgia is a real — and treatable — condition.

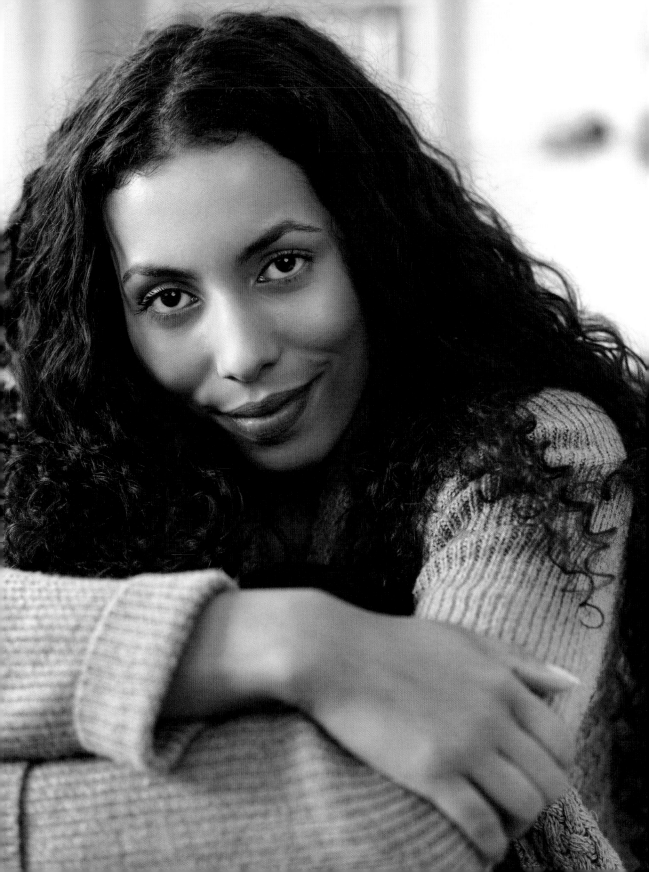

CHAPTER 3

Myths vs. facts

It's no secret that fibromyalgia has a credibility problem. Just take an informal poll among friends or do a quick search on the internet. From average people on the street to doctors who've been practicing medicine for years, some truly understand fibromyalgia, while others don't know much about it.

To help move you forward in your understanding of fibromyalgia, this chapter outlines several myths about the condition and uncovers the truth behind each one.

SOLVING A MYSTERY

In Chapter 2, you read about the history of fibromyalgia. You also learned about how things have changed over the years in terms of what's known about it.

Fibromyalgia is still fairly young in terms of what is known about it. After all, the word *fibromyalgia* has been around only since

1976, and it wasn't officially defined until the 1990s. With that said, fibromyalgia tends to provoke many questions.

Your doctor may wonder: *How can you tell the difference between fibromyalgia and a different condition, such as arthritis or depression? These symptoms are all over the place. What tests should I order for this patient? What's the best treatment to advise?*

At the same time, you may be wondering: *Will I ever feel better? What damage is this doing to my body? Am I going to have this for the rest of my life? What's wrong with me?*

A lot of research has been done on fibromyalgia since it was first recognized by the American College of Rheumatology in 1990. Even so, answering questions like these takes time.

Chances are, you didn't know many, if any, other people who had fibromyalgia before learning you have it. Even today, fibromyalgia is a condition that's still largely unrecognized. Medical professionals are at all different points along the learning curve.

Fibromyalgia is a challenging mystery. It can be seen as a whodunit of sorts — or maybe more of a "whatdunit." Although many people love good mysteries, most people also love to solve them. In the interest of "solving" fibromyalgia, here's a look at the many theories floating around about it. What follows are the most common myths about fibromyalgia and the truths behind them.

Myth 1. Fibromyalgia isn't real

This is the top misconception about fibromyalgia. People sometimes think that fibromyalgia isn't a real medical problem or that it's "all in your head." Fibromyalgia symptoms can be so vague that they could apply to any number of conditions. Plus, who hasn't felt sore, tired or moody — or all of those things at once — on a regular basis?

Truth: Many, if not most, medical illnesses aren't seen as real until more is known about them. At one point, even asthma was thought to be a made-up condition. Rheumatoid arthritis was once thought to be an infection. In both cases, knowing more about how they developed led to better understanding, as well as better ways to diagnose and treat them. Fibromyalgia has been — and in some circles, is still — in the same situation. More pieces of the puzzle are coming together every day.

Bottom line: Fibromyalgia is caused by a real problem happening within the body. It's thought to be caused by a glitch in how the brain and nerves throughout the spinal cord process pain signals. As a result, people with fibromyalgia react more strongly to pain and many other sensations.

Myth 2. Fibromyalgia is a mental health disorder

Fibromyalgia can be hard to diagnose. When one test after another comes back with no solid answers, some doctors may wonder if a patient's symptoms are actually related to a mental health condition, instead of something that's physically happening in the body.

Truth: While symptoms of fibromyalgia may be *related* to things going on in your mind, such as stress and depression, fibromyalgia itself isn't in your head. Fibromyalgia is a medical disorder, not a mental health disorder. And it isn't caused by a mental health disorder, although you'll learn in this book that stress can play a role in your symptoms and in fibromyalgia in general.

It's also important to note that having any kind of medical condition can make a person feel anxious or depressed. If you feel frustrated that you have a chronic condition that seems to get in the way of everything, you aren't alone.

Bottom line: Fibromyalgia is a real, physical condition. It's caused by a miscommunication between the nerves in your body and your brain. (Learn more on page 47.)

Myth 3. Fibromyalgia is an autoimmune disorder

Autoimmune disorders affect more than 23 million people in the U.S., and they can involve nearly any part of the body, inside and out.

It's your autoimmune system's job to fight off viruses and bacteria before they make you sick. When you have an autoimmune

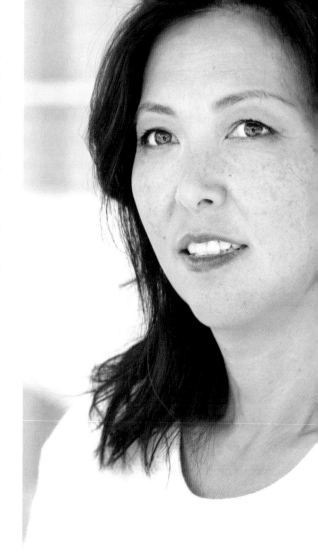
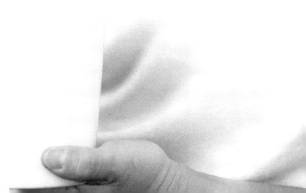

disorder, your immune system mistakenly attacks healthy cells instead. There are more than 80 conditions labeled as autoimmune disorders. Some common ones are rheumatoid arthritis, Hashimoto's disease, celiac disease and lupus. Fibromyalgia isn't on the list. Here's why.

Truth: The idea that the body can turn against itself has been around only since the turn of the 20th century. Around the same time, experts were trying to better understand fibromyalgia — known as fibrositis back then. At that time, what would eventually be called fibromyalgia was placed in the same category as rheumatoid arthritis. It was labeled as an autoimmune disorder. Doctors would learn later on that about 1 in 4 people with fibromyalgia also has an autoimmune disorder. This finding led to fibromyalgia remaining lumped together with autoimmune disorders.

But fibromyalgia isn't an autoimmune disorder. Fibromyalgia and autoimmune disorders — and many other conditions, for that matter — often share many symptoms. Joint and muscle pain, swelling, muscle weakness, and fatigue are all examples. But the blood tests used to diagnose autoimmune disorders aren't used to diagnose fibromyalgia. Plus, a physical exam is often enough for a doctor to be able to tell if you have an autoimmune disorder or fibromyalgia.

Put simply, they're two different types of conditions. That also means that medications used to treat an autoimmune disorder can't address symptoms of fibromyalgia.

One more difference between autoimmune disorders and fibromyalgia: Autoimmune disorders often cause permanent damage in the body, including to skin and joints. Fibromyalgia doesn't damage your body.

Bottom line: Although fibromyalgia can occur along with an autoimmune disorder, fibromyalgia itself isn't an autoimmune disorder. Researchers are studying what links these disorders together, but they are separate and distinct disorders.

Myth 4. Fibromyalgia is a connective tissue disorder

Cartilage, bones and fat are types of connective tissue. They create a sturdy web of proteins that supports your body and gives it strength. Without connective tissue, your body would be floppy and shapeless.

Connective tissue disorders can change how parts of your body look and grow. They can affect your skin, bones, joints, organs, blood vessels, eyes and ears. They can also change the way your tissues work. More than 200 disorders can affect your connective tissue. Some may be inherited from your parents, while others are types of cancer or autoimmune disorders. Autoimmune connective tissue disorders cause your immune system to attack your body's supportive framework.

There are two different types of connective tissue disorders: connective tissue disorders that are present at birth and autoimmune connective tissue disorders. Autoimmune connective tissue disorders cause your immune system to attack your body's supportive framework and organs. Connective tissue disorders that are present at birth include Ehlers-Danlos syndrome and Marfan syndrome. These disorders cause the joints, tendons and muscles to be unusually flexible. This can cause the joints to get dislocated, among other problems.

In the early 1800s, fibromyalgia — then called muscular rheumatism — was thought of as a connective tissue disorder. That's because a Scottish surgeon found knots of fibrous tissue in the muscles and connective tissues of people who had conditions such as rheumatoid arthritis and lupus. Rheumatoid arthritis and lupus are autoimmune connective tissue disorders, so it was thought that the swelling and irritation that came with connective tissue disorders were causing fibromyalgia.

One hundred years later, fibromyalgia had a different name — fibrositis. Although it had a new name, experts still had the same thought — that fibromyalgia resulted from swelling and irritation. Eventually, scientists at Mayo Clinic studied samples of tissue from people who had fibrositis. They found no inflammation at all.

Truth: To date, no one has been able to find proof of swelling and irritation in the tissues of people who have fibromyalgia. The name of the condition even reflects the fact that fibromyalgia isn't caused by swelling and irritation in the body's tissues. While it used to be called fibrositis ("-itis" means swelling and irritation), today, it's called fibromyalgia ("-algia" means pain). Its name indicates that it's a pain disorder, not a connective tissue disorder.

Connective tissue disorders can get confused with fibromyalgia because the two conditions can happen together. And some symptoms of the two types of disorders overlap, such as pain and tiredness. But they aren't the same type of condition.

If you have a connective tissue disorder, a blood test will likely reveal proteins or markers showing inflammation in your body. These same blood tests come back normal for someone with fibromyalgia.

Bottom line: While even today some people still think that fibromyalgia is a connective tissue disorder, the fact is that it's not. Put simply, fibromyalgia is a pain disorder.

Myth 5. You're just looking for attention

Many people don't understand fibromyalgia. Unless you have it or have a loved one who has it, it can be hard to understand what it means to live with fibromyalgia day in and day out. If you have fibromyalgia, you've probably run into people who say, "You don't look sick," "That's all you talk about," or "Oh, that's nothing. At least you don't have … " Sometimes even people who care can unintentionally make comments that hurt.

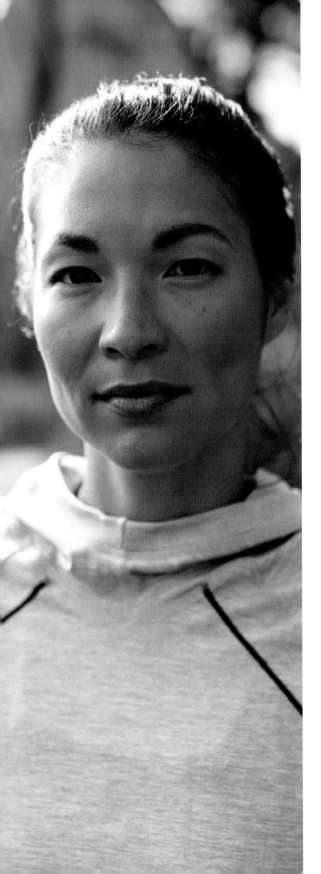

For a number of reasons, people may react to your fibromyalgia as though you're seeking attention. Many people have only a passing knowledge about fibromyalgia, if they know anything about it at all.

Truth: Research shows that only 1 in 4 graduating primary care doctors feels capable of helping patients manage chronic pain. In light of this, you may not learn about treatments from your doctor that can help you feel better. And if you're constantly talking to a doctor who doesn't understand fibromyalgia — or maybe doesn't believe it exists — you may end up feeling as if you're looking for attention when all you really want is understanding and to feel better.

Bottom line: First, be patient with yourself. It can be tough to feel as if you're surrounded by skeptical people. Next, be patient with others. This may seem like a tall order when you're feeling hurt and misunderstood. Know that doctors and loved ones want to help — they just may not always know how.

Try to find moments when you can share what you've learned about fibromyalgia with your loved ones and people on your health care team. This can help all of you move forward in understanding fibromyalgia and how its symptoms are affecting you.

Myth 6. You're a hypochondriac

Over the years, it's been thought that fibromyalgia was made up by a stressed-out,

"KNOW THAT DOCTORS AND LOVED ONES WANT TO HELP – THEY MAY JUST NOT ALWAYS KNOW HOW."

overtaxed mind and the result of being a hypochondriac. This is in part because people with fibromyalgia often go from doctor to doctor only to be told there's nothing wrong with them.

Truth: Despite their seeming similarities, fibromyalgia and hypochondriasis (also called hypochondria) are two separate entities. Hypochondriasis starts in the mind, while fibromyalgia has a physical cause. A hypochondriac constantly worries that he or she has an illness even though nothing is wrong. If you're a hypochondriac, you may believe your symptoms are the result of a severe disease, even though test after test doesn't show that anything's wrong.

Hypochondriasis and its symptoms are most often mentally induced, meaning that they start in the mind. Fibromyalgia symptoms, on the other hand, stem from a problem with the way the brain processes pain signals and other physical sensations.

Bottom line: With both fibromyalgia and hypochondriasis, test after test comes back normal, so you may be able to see how people can confuse the two. But you're not a hypochondriac. A better way to describe what you're feeling may be health anxiety.

Myth 7. You're just lazy

Take a look in a mirror. Do you look like you have fibromyalgia? Probably not. You likely look the same as you always have. Other people see you the same way: You look fine from the outside. So people who don't know much about fibromyalgia may think you're lazy when you cancel plans, withdraw from them or often aren't at work. That's because if you look fine, you must feel fine, too. They may think that you use fibromyalgia to avoid things that you don't want to do — in effect, that you're lazy.

Truth: When it comes to fibromyalgia, what people *don't* see is what matters. They didn't see you this morning struggling to stretch and flex your stiff limbs, trying to guess how achy you'll feel today. They didn't see the debate you had with yourself before you even got out of bed: *I am exhausted and really don't feel like doing this again today … just a little more time under the covers. But I can't stay in bed forever. If I don't work, I won't be able to pay the bills.*

Without treatment, fibromyalgia can make it hard to work and take part in everyday activities. Any one of its core symptoms — chronic widespread pain, fatigue, trouble sleeping, anxiety, depression — would be enough to make an otherwise healthy person call in sick for the day. From there, these effects trickle down into all aspects of your life. To someone who doesn't understand the effects of fibromyalgia, you may be seen as lazy or unmotivated — but this couldn't be further from the truth.

Bottom line: Many people with fibromyalgia search tirelessly for answers to find out what's wrong with them and how to feel better. They're quite motivated and more than willing to put in the work that's needed to win their daily battle with their bodies. That's anything but lazy.

Myth 8. You're just stressed

It's common to get stressed out now and then. Stress is a normal reaction to what happens in life, whether it's good or bad — such as a new job or the death of a loved one. Depending on who you are and what's going on in your life, when you're faced with stress, you may sail through the choppy waters, you may spin in circles without a paddle, or you may do a little of both.

Whether it's mild or severe, stress can affect your health even without your realizing it. You may think illness is to blame for your nagging headache, being unable to sleep or being less productive at work.

But stress may be the culprit. Stress can affect your body, your thoughts and feelings, and your behavior.

Because fibromyalgia and stress share so many symptoms, it's likely that you could be feeling stress and not have fibromyalgia, right? Not so fast.

Truth: Although stress and fibromyalgia have many symptoms in common, they can differ in how long they last and how severe they are. For example, stress can cause tense muscles. But the muscle pain of fibromyalgia often is described as a constant, dull ache that has lasted for at least three months. And while you may feel pain when you're stressed, the pain of fibromyalgia is widespread. That means it affects both sides of the body, above and below the waist.

Sleep is another example of how stress and fibromyalgia differ. Stress can cause you to not feel well and feel tired during the day. But in fibromyalgia, sleep problems and fatigue are more severe. People who have fibromyalgia often say they feel tired as soon as they awaken, even after sleeping for long periods of time.

Bottom line: Researchers are studying what links stress and fibromyalgia, but they are separate and distinct. At first glance, the symptoms of the two can look a lot alike. But are they one and the same? Not at all. However, they are linked. Stress plays a major role in the story of fibromyalgia, often appearing as a key player from the start.

You'll learn more about stress in fibromyalgia in Chapter 15. For now, it's important to know that stress and fibromyalgia are different. However, the same strategies that can relieve stress can also help with fibromyalgia. Stress relievers you can do on your own include:

- Trying mind-body exercises, such as meditation, yoga or deep breathing
- Getting regular physical activity
- Getting enough sleep
- Eating a healthy diet
- Managing your time

One of the best reasons to tackle stress is the fact that stress may be what sets fibromyalgia in motion for you. Research shows that stress triggers fibromyalgia in about 5 to 10 percent of people with the condition.

While stress and fibromyalgia are clearly linked, their close relationship is only an association of two separate conditions that share a lot in common and may affect each other on a regular basis.

Myth 9. You're just depressed

Similar to stress, depression often occurs right alongside fibromyalgia. Does this mean that if you think you have fibromyalgia, depression may be what's causing your symptoms?

Truth: While depression and fibromyalgia may look alike, they're different. Each has its own causes and treatment options.

Depression doesn't cause fibromyalgia. But research suggests that depression may make it more likely that you'll develop fibromyalgia. Plus, the effects of having a chronic con-

dition may cause you to feel depressed. A chronic condition like fibromyalgia can cause loss and limitations that could certainly lead to depression. And any person with a life-altering medical condition can get depressed. Think for a moment about someone you know who has or had cancer. It probably wouldn't surprise you if that person was depressed. You would never tell that person that being in a better mood would make the cancer go away, right? The same can be said for someone who has fibromyalgia.

Bottom line: Depression can be treated, and for people who have fibromyalgia, it's especially important to do so. Together, these disorders are exhausting mentally and physically. Treating depression frees up energy you can use to cope with the challenges of fibromyalgia.

Myth 10. Fibromyalgia isn't there if no test or X-ray can prove it

In a fast-paced world of instant answers and easy solutions, fibromyalgia offers neither. This doesn't sit well with some people. Fibromyalgia can't be easily confirmed or ruled out through a simple lab test. Your doctor can't detect it in your blood or see it on an X-ray. Because there's no test for fibromyalgia, your doctor must rely on your group of symptoms to say for sure if you have it. Because pain and other symptoms can vary from person to person, some people find that this method isn't scientific enough to pass muster.

Truth: Fibromyalgia isn't the only condition that doctors have a hard time diagnosing. Doctors have to rely on a person's symptoms to diagnose a whole host of conditions, including migraine, depression, irritable bowel syndrome, chronic fatigue syndrome, other pain disorders, and a variety of pelvic and bladder pain syndromes. Each of these conditions lacks an objective test that can say for sure if someone has it. As with fibromyalgia, doctors diagnose these disorders by ruling out other conditions first.

For fibromyalgia, doctors generally use a set of criteria created by experts who have vast experience in treating people who have the condition. However, because symptoms often overlap with those of other conditions, making a firm diagnosis takes patience and determination for everyone involved.

There may be new tests on the horizon, though. Advanced imaging tests of the brain are starting to show researchers what the brain looks like in someone who has fibromyalgia. This research, paired with newer imaging machines, may be able to show more detail about the brain, including how it responds to pain and changes in chemicals that affect the pain experience. Newer technology also may one day be able to show abnormalities that can point to fibromyalgia symptoms, such as slower brain function and mental fogginess.

Bottom line: As more study is done that may one day lead to a faster way to diagnose fibromyalgia, researchers have learned

a lot. They've learned that changes in the central nervous system cause changes in how pain is processed. They also know that changes in the brain are what cause many of the symptoms of fibromyalgia.

Myth 11. Only middle-aged women get fibromyalgia

It's true that middle-aged women are far more likely to develop fibromyalgia. However, it strikes both men and women and people of all ages.

Truth: The National Institute of Arthritis and Musculoskeletal and Skin Diseases notes that between 80 to 90 percent of people diagnosed with fibromyalgia are women. This means that between 1 and 2 out of every 10 people who have fibromyalgia *are not* women.

And fibromyalgia doesn't always affect men and women in the same way. Men often have fewer symptoms, fewer pain sites, less-frequent fatigue, less-frequent irritable bowel syndrome, and fewer tender points. This knowledge helped lead to new criteria to improve how fibromyalgia is diagnosed. For example, tender points are no longer required for a fibromyalgia diagnosis. The criteria that's used today is based on a range of symptoms. In turn, more men are being diagnosed with the condition.

Similar to its impact on women, fibromyalgia has a heavy impact on men's physical health, mental well-being, relationships and careers. But research shows that there's a difference between how men and women with fibromyalgia are viewed. Traditionally, for example, men are expected to be tougher. This can lead to a lack of understanding among close family and friends and in the workplace. Plus, many doctors still see fibromyalgia as a disease that only affects women. As more men are diagnosed, it will take time for peoples' views on fibromyalgia to change.

As is the case with men, children and adolescents aren't typically seen as being affected by fibromyalgia. While it's true that fibromyalgia is usually seen in people between the ages of 30 and 60, younger people can have it, too. A child may have symptoms that go unrecognized until adulthood.

Estimates suggest that fibromyalgia affects 2 to 6 percent of school children, mostly girls. It's most commonly diagnosed between ages 13 and 15. Children with fibromyalgia have the same symptoms as do adults. This can seriously affect their school experience and relationships with peers.

Bottom line: Although women may be diagnosed with fibromyalgia more often, it's a disorder that can affect anyone of any age or any ethnicity.

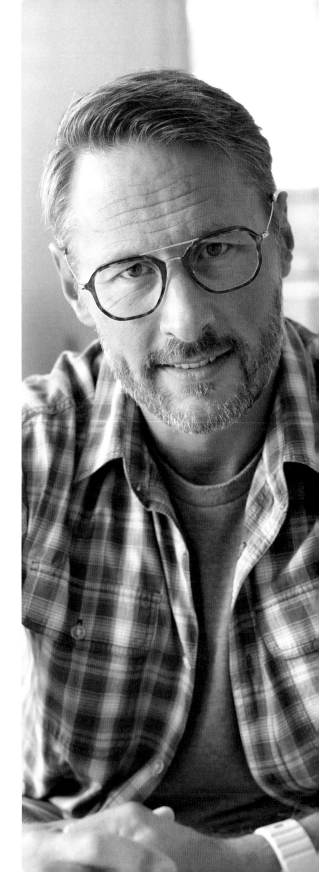

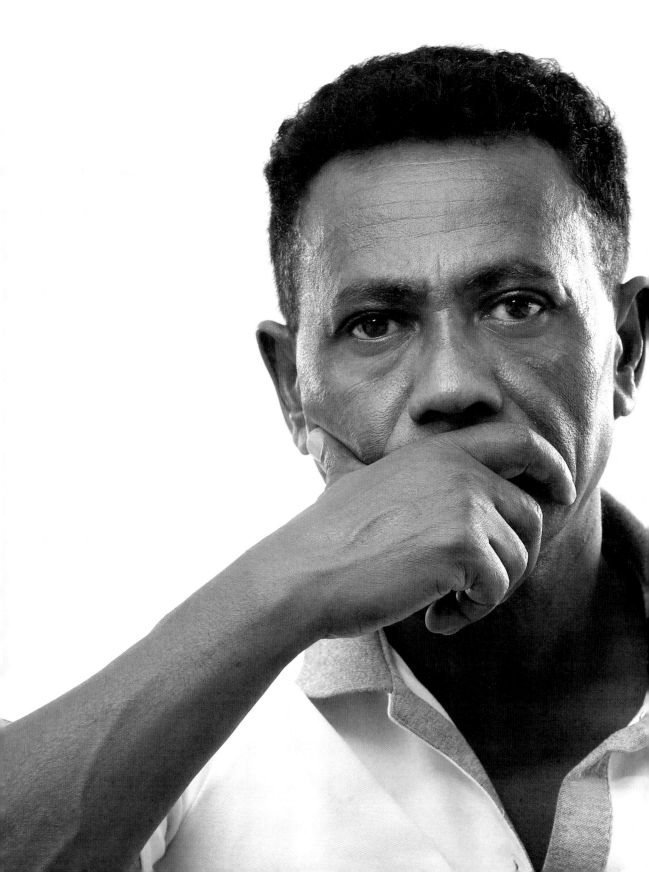

CHAPTER 4

What causes fibromyalgia?

If you have fibromyalgia, it's natural to want to know why you have this condition. What caused it to happen? Could it have been prevented? Why are you feeling so many different things, aside from pain? What is happening in your body?

The "why" behind fibromyalgia is still under study. But medical experts and researchers know more about it now than they ever have. This chapter offers the latest insights into what happens in the body to cause fibromyalgia. Among these insights, you'll read about a disorder called central sensitization. You'll learn why researchers and medical experts believe that this disorder is what leads to fibromyalgia in the first place.

With all of this said, keep in mind that although knowing the *why* behind fibromyalgia is helpful, it's even more important to know *how* to manage it. This chapter offers answers to many questions you may be asking — and that's one more step toward managing your symptoms and living a full, enjoyable life.

WHY DO I HAVE FIBROMYALGIA?

If you've been diagnosed with fibromyalgia, the path that's led you there may have been a frustrating one. Even today, you may still feel that you have more questions than you have answers. You may also still be

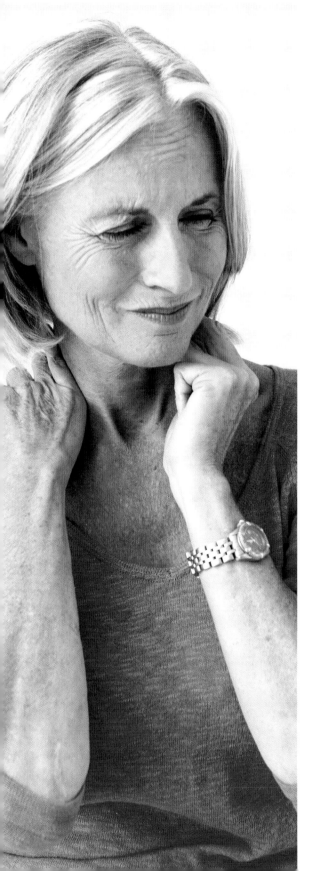

seeking relief from the pain and other symptoms you're experiencing.

You've likely undergone a number of tests to rule out other medical conditions. If that's the case, it's also likely that those test results haven't given you much — if any — new information, other than to tell you about all of the conditions that you *don't* have. All of this stems from the fact that no single test can tell you that you have fibromyalgia. As you'll learn in Chapter 5, diagnosing fibromyalgia has changed over the years and takes several different steps.

To add to this, you may have felt as if your family, friends or even members of your health care team didn't believe you when you first told them what you've been feeling. Maybe you've been told that it's all in your mind, or any number of other myths that you learned about in Chapter 3. All the while, the pain that no one can explain remains, and nothing you do seems to make it any better. Things that shouldn't hurt, such as a gentle touch, do hurt, and pain seems be more intense than it should.

All of this may be leaving you feeling stressed and unsure about your future.

Although more is known about fibromyalgia today, this condition is still under study. As researchers continue to work on piecing together its puzzle of symptoms, this much is known:
• Fibromyalgia is a long-term health condition. It impacts the central nervous system, affecting how the brain processes

pain. Widespread pain, fatigue, sleep issues and lapses in memory are just some of its symptoms.
- Fibromyalgia isn't progressive, meaning it's not a condition that gets worse over time. Fibromyalgia is also not life-threatening, and it won't damage your joints, muscles or nerves.

Researchers have also learned that a number of conditions and events may trigger the onset of fibromyalgia. In people with fibromyalgia, any one of these can have a dramatic effect on the body — particularly, on the nervous system.

Research also shows that some health conditions that affect the joints, muscles and bones may be linked to fibromyalgia. They include osteoarthritis, rheumatoid arthritis, lupus and a form of arthritis that mostly affects the spine (ankylosing spondylitis).

The good news is that in recent years, researchers have been digging deeper to learn more about what happens in the body during fibromyalgia. They've learned that a disorder known as central sensitization may be at play.

What is central sensitization?

Many chronic pain conditions, including fibromyalgia, can be traced to the central nervous system — the brain and spinal cord in particular. Here's why this is important.

Your body is covered in sensor cells. These cells keep track of what's going on with your body. For example, they monitor what you feel, taste, touch or smell. These cells send the information they gather to your spinal cord. From there, the information travels up to your brain.

OTHER CONDITIONS CAUSED BY CENTRAL SENSITIZATION

Aside from pain, many other symptoms and syndromes have been linked to central sensitization. Several are also seen in fibromyalgia.

- Numbness or tingling
- Headaches, both migraine and tension
- Irritable bowel syndrome (IBS)
- Chronic fatigue syndrome
- Positional orthostatic tachycardia syndrome (POTS)
- Interstitial cystitis
- Restless legs syndrome
- Temporomandibular joint (TMJ) disorder
- Sleep problems
- Dizziness or lightheadedness
- Brain fog, including memory problems and a short attention span
- Depression or anxiety
- Weakness
- Sensitivity to light, noise, food, medication or changes in the environment
- Nerve pain

When your brain receives the information from your sensor cells, it decides what to do with that information. Too hot? Find some shade. Too cold? Turn up the heat. Thirsty? Get a drink of water. These are all examples of decisions that the brain tells you to make after it sorts through the information that these tiny cells send.

But with central sensitization, this communication gets turned up, much like the volume on your radio. Over time, the brain starts to think that ordinary sensations, such as a light touch, hurt, even though they normally wouldn't. It's as if your sensors are on high alert, all sending out screams for help to your brain even though there's no true emergency. In turn, a nervous system that's in a constant state of high alert over a period of time causes everything you feel to get turned up, too.

If you have fibromyalgia, think for a moment about the many symptoms you're experiencing. Central sensitization — in other words, a "turned-up" nervous system —

explains how you can be feeling so many different things, maybe all at the same time, and how they all can be affecting you so deeply. This is what experts believe causes the variety of symptoms related to fibromyalgia — pain, numbness and tingling, mental fogginess, dizziness, sleep problems, fatigue, and others.

Other ways pain messages get to the brain The brain and spinal cord are two major players in central sensitization. But other culprits can contribute to overzealous pain messages, too.

For example, part of your nervous system connects your brain and spinal cord to other parts of your body (peripheral nervous system). The nerves in this system take messages from your muscles and organs and send them to your brain. Damage to these nerves can cause miscommunication about pain to reach the brain.

Chemical changes in the brain also can be to blame. Put simply, chemicals play a role in getting messages from the rest of your body to your brain. You may have too few or too many of these chemicals, known as neurotransmitters, and this can affect how and what messages are sent to your brain from other parts of your body.

Medication also can affect the chemicals that are already naturally in your body. If, for example, your doctor prescribes medications to treat your symptoms, they introduce more chemicals into your body. When they get together, these medications can cause a sort of chemical confusion that can change what — and how many — pain messages get to your brain. This chemical confusion can make pain worse.

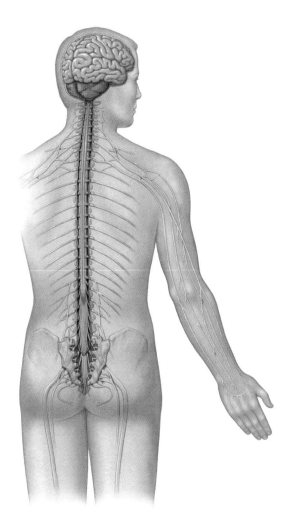

The peripheral nervous system connects your brain and spinal cord to other parts of your body. The nerves in this system take messages from your muscles and organs and send them to your brain.

What causes fibromyalgia?   49

Inside the brain Going back to the brain, you've already learned that fibromyalgia is thought to be caused by changes in how the brain handles the messages it receives. That's the idea behind central sensitization. But other changes also happen in the brain.

With the help of a research technique called dynamic magnetic resonance imaging, researchers have compared the brains of people experiencing central sensitization against the brains of those who aren't. In people with this disorder, experts can see that more of the brain lights up in response to pain. In other words, it's as though the areas of the brain that are supposed to process pain are working — but they're asking other areas of the brain to focus on pain, too. That means that in people who have this disorder, more of the brain is paying attention to pain.

At the same time, the pathways and connections within the brain are more direct. Picture a map with a mix of large highways and small, rural roads and side streets. This is how the brain's connections are typically mapped out. But with central sensitization and in fibromyalgia, few small roads and side streets exist. Instead, the map is overtaken by a few large highways, all designed to carry the load of extra pain messages from all over the body to the brain.

This leads to a concept known as neuroplasticity. Neuroplasticity describes how your brain changes over time when you learn new things, experience changes or adapt to the world around you. This is usually a good thing. But in central sensitization, it isn't. Instead, it's as though no one shut off the light switch — or in this case, your nerves — that are telling your brain about the pain or other symptoms you've experienced. Pain from an injury, for example, may have long since resolved, but no one told your nerves this. They're still firing off messages to your brain about it, as though the pain is still there. That creates ongoing pain and related symptoms and keeps those messages traveling to your brain, causing you to feel them over and over again. This leads to pain and other symptoms getting worse and worse over time.

WHAT ELSE DOES RESEARCH SHOW?

Although central sensitization is one theory behind the cause of fibromyalgia, researchers are studying other possible causes as well. Here are some of the latest findings.

Whiplash and other forms of physical trauma

Studying people who have fibromyalgia, some experts have found that as many as half can trace the onset of their symptoms to one event that involved trauma or injury.

For example, researchers studied people with a whiplash injury after a car accident and found that 1 in 5 had symptoms related to the injury a full two years later. Participants reported ongoing fatigue, headaches, anxiety, and sensitivity to light and sound. The researchers thought that the pain from the injury may have spread to other parts of the nervous system, causing pain in other parts of the body, as well as additional symptoms. While this may be one illustration of how trauma can lead to fibromyalgia, other researchers haven't been able to confirm these findings. More study on the link between a whiplash injury and fibromyalgia is needed.

Chemical exposures, disorders such as lupus or rheumatoid arthritis, and serious infections, such as mononucleosis, also fall under the category of physical trauma that can lead to fibromyalgia. Some people with fibromyalgia say that they got sick and never felt like they fully recovered from it.

Sleep disorders

Sleep disorders are common with fibromyalgia. People who have fibromyalgia often have problems falling asleep and staying asleep, and they often don't feel rested, no matter how long they sleep. Sleep that's not restful and restorative is a hallmark of fibromyalgia, and it can lead to other symptoms, including fatigue and brain fog.

Mood disorders and emotional trauma

Mood disorders are a delicate subject in fibromyalgia. For many years, as you learned earlier in this book (see Chapter 2), doctors thought that people who reported having

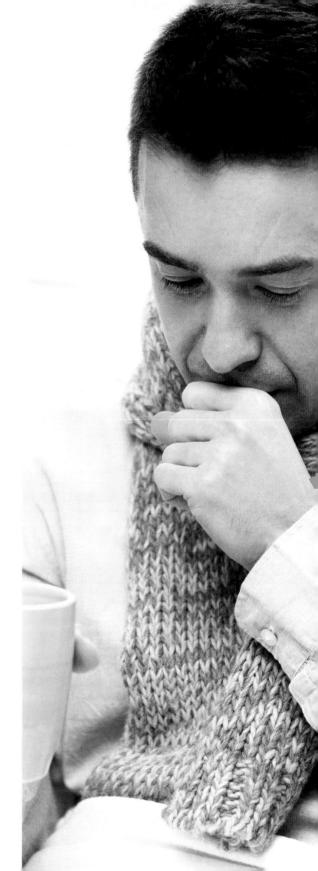

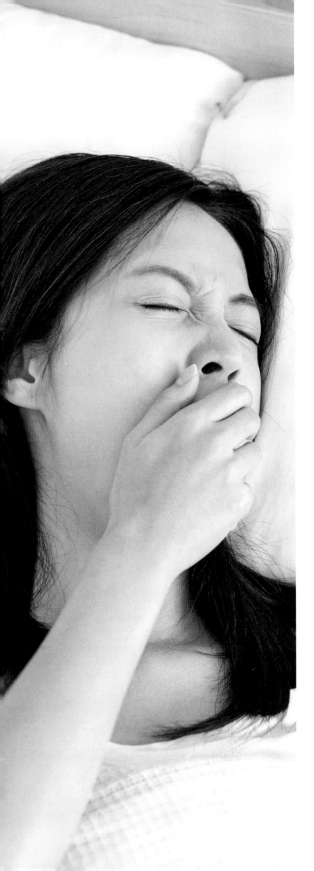

symptoms of fibromyalgia were making them up because they couldn't find a cause to explain them. Today, health care professionals know that depression and anxiety are real symptoms of fibromyalgia — but these mood disorders may actually cause fibromyalgia, too.

Some studies show that fibromyalgia tends to be more common in families that also have a history of mood disorders and anxiety. It's also known that depression, anxiety and other mood disorders add stress to the body. This can sometimes lead to fibromyalgia and can make symptoms worse.

Mood disorders and emotional trauma, even when they're experienced early in life, can also lead to fibromyalgia. Post-traumatic stress disorder (PTSD) can also affect the way people respond to stress and can affect how well someone copes with pain. Researchers have found that experiences of emotional trauma and post-traumatic stress can lead to symptoms of fibromyalgia.

HOW AND WHY YOU FEEL PAIN

Now that you know a little more about what causes fibromyalgia, how does this translate into the pain you're likely feeling?

You already know that pain is one of the hallmark symptoms of fibromyalgia. Some people describe it as a constant, dull ache throughout the body that never seems to go away. The pain is chronic — that means that it's pain that doesn't go away for three

"CHOICES YOU MAKE DAY TO DAY CAN HELP YOU ... IMPROVE YOUR QUALITY OF LIFE."

months or longer. This is different from acute pain, which is meant to protect you when your body is damaged by an injury, for example. Chronic pain may or may not have an obvious cause, and as you've learned in this chapter, it can stick around even after you've healed from an injury or surgery, for example.

This pain can be mild or extreme, and you may feel more pain some days than others. How much pain you feel may even change throughout the day. It may affect your joints or your muscles. You may not know what's causing the pain, and often, there's no inflammation involved, like there is with other pain-related conditions.

You learned earlier in this chapter that in fibromyalgia, your nervous system gets "turned up" and even re-routed. The sensors throughout your body are interpreting various sensations as pain and sending those messages up to your brain. In turn, more and more of the messages getting sent to your brain are pain related. From there, more of your nervous system is dedicated to feelings of pain.

In short, this is how chronic pain can get worse and worse over time in fibromyalgia.

Changing the pain experience

You're learning in Part 1 of this book what fibromyalgia is, what it isn't and what's happening in your body. While this is important background to have, keep in mind that you have the power to change this scenario. Choices you make day to day can help you manage the symptoms you're feeling and improve your quality of life. You don't have to live a life that's constantly full of pain and other symptoms that may be limiting you now. While certain symptoms are a reality of fibromyalgia, you can choose how much of a reality they are for you.

You'll learn much more about this later in this book. Ultimately, you'll create a daily plan you can start using right away. But for now, reflecting on what you've learned in this chapter may help you start to see ways that you can improve how you're feeling.

In this chapter, you've learned about what causes fibromyalgia and how the symptoms you're feeling are linked to changes in your body that happen with this condition. With fibromyalgia, pain and other symptoms take over your nervous system so that their messages are the loudest — the ones that your brain is hearing most.

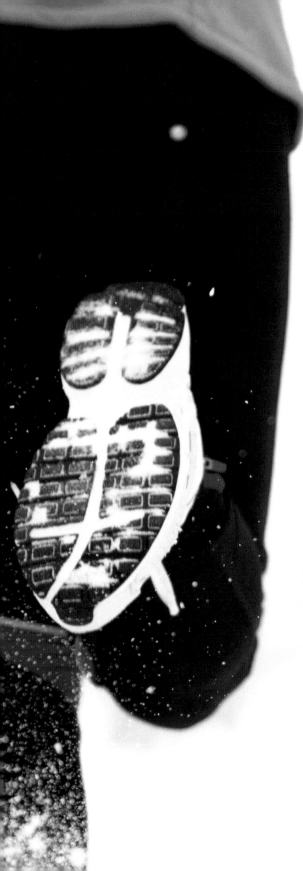

Your pain pathways shout their messages so loudly that they drown out other messages about experiences that are more pleasant. Eventually, it's almost as though your brain isn't hearing about anything else but pain and discomfort.

What if you could reverse this trend? Think for a moment about changing the pathways in your nervous system and the messages that get to your brain. What if you could create more pathways that tell your brain about other, more enjoyable experiences? In turn, could you make the pathways that are constantly shouting about pain to your brain get quieter and quieter? The short answer is yes. You have the power to make this happen.

You'll learn how to do this as you read through the rest of this book. But you can start thinking about this now by asking yourself this question: *How do you react to your pain?*

In this chapter, you've learned that fibromyalgia is caused by changes in the nervous system that lead to an overcommunication to your brain about pain and other discomfort. How you react to pain can either strengthen the pain messages that your brain hears — or make them quieter.

Here's an example: On days when your pain is worse, how do you react? Do you choose to avoid physical activity until you're feeling better? If you said yes, know that this is a normal instinct. Many people with fibromyalgia react in the same way.

But this response actually isn't the best choice. Doing less when you're in pain will actually make your pain worse. Why is this?

First, if you avoid activity when you're in pain, you may do too much when you're feeling better. This, in turn, can lead to more pain. Second, inactivity will make your muscles weaker over time. This will make it harder to do things with less effort — and with less pain. Pacing and moderating your activity no matter how you're feeling on any given day is a better choice than avoiding activity completely. Plus, physical activity helps quiet the pain signals that are reaching your brain.

You'll learn more about physical activity in Chapter 13 and pacing and moderation in Chapter 14.

A reason for hope

Not knowing the exact cause of your fibromyalgia symptoms can certainly be disheartening and frustrating at times. But as you've learned in this chapter, progress has been made in understanding why and how fibromyalgia happens. This, alone, is a reason for hope.

Knowing more about the how and the why behind this condition offers a starting point on a road map toward effectively managing it and living a fulfilling, enjoyable life.

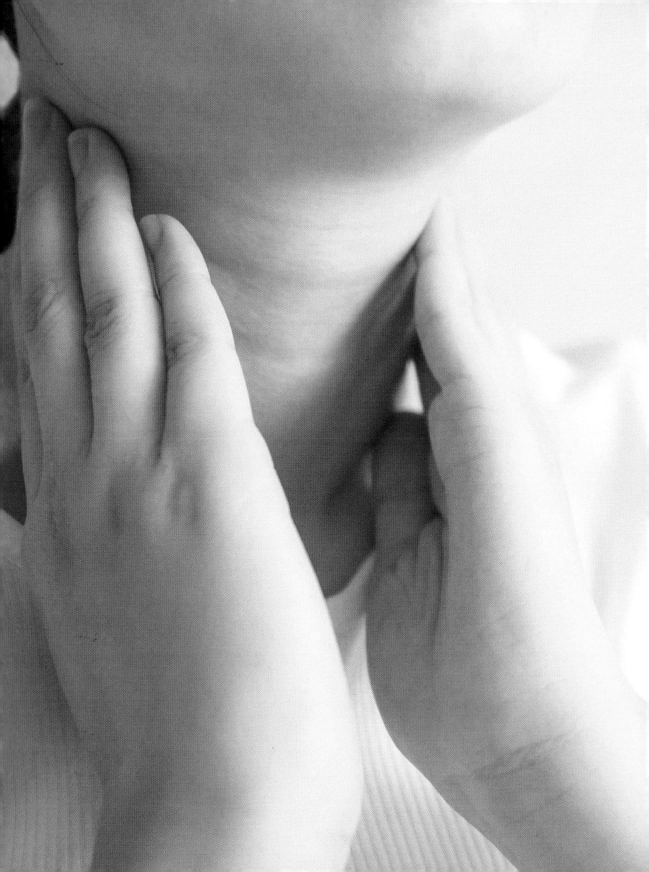

CHAPTER 5

How do I know
if I have fibromyalgia?

Some people with fibromyalgia say that their pain feels like a dull ache all over their body. Others say that they feel as if they have the flu and can't shake it. If someone asks what fibromyalgia feels like for you, you may say that you're always tired. Or maybe you don't feel as though you can get a good night's sleep. Or, you may say that it's hard to focus or remember things. You may describe fibromyalgia as all of this and more — everyone's experience with fibromyalgia is different.

With this said, how do you know if what you're experiencing is fibromyalgia or something else entirely? In this chapter, you'll learn about how doctors diagnose fibromyalgia and how that process has changed over time. You'll also find out which symptoms are thought to be a part of fibromyalgia.

NOT EASY TO DIAGNOSE

It may not come as a surprise that fibromyalgia is hard for doctors to diagnose. Its symptoms can overlap with those of other disorders. It's also not uncommon for people who have fibromyalgia to have other medical conditions. This can muddy the waters even more. Plus, the range of symptoms can vary wildly from one person to another.

There's no one test that can say for sure if you have fibromyalgia. However, experts have learned that fibromyalgia has a certain signature that can help doctors diagnose it with accuracy. The process starts with gathering your medical history, learning about your symptoms and conducting a physical exam that includes a number of blood tests. Other tests may be done to rule out other possible disorders.

This is often the process doctors take today to diagnose fibromyalgia. However, it's taken decades to get to this point.

HOW MAKING A DIAGNOSIS HAS CHANGED

Fibromyalgia has a long history, dating back thousands of years.

Although many advances were made over the years, it wasn't until 1990 that the World Health Organization recognized fibromyalgia as an official disorder. And it wasn't long before that — in 1976 — that this disorder was given the name it has today. Before then, doctors couldn't find a physical cause for fibromyalgia, so they often mislabeled it as a mental health disorder.

Although there's still no one test that can reveal fibromyalgia as the cause of someone's symptoms, there are tests that can be done. The results of these tests can help doctors determine if someone has fibromyalgia or not. Here's how this process has changed over the years, leading to how fibromyalgia is diagnosed today.

1990 guidelines

The American College of Rheumatology released the first guidelines for fibromyalgia in 1990. These guidelines made doctors more aware of the disorder. They also helped doctors see more easily when someone had symptoms that lined up with the condition. According to these guidelines, people were said to have fibromyalgia if they had:
1. Widespread, chronic pain that lasted for at least three months.

WHAT DOES "WIDESPREAD PAIN" MEAN?

The term "widespread pain" is common to fibromyalgia. It describes pain in certain areas of your body, along pathways that lead to your brain. Widespread pain is pain that you feel in both the left and the right sides of your body, in areas above and below your waist.

WHAT ARE TENDER POINTS?

The first set of guidelines for diagnosing fibromyalgia required testing of tender points all over the body. When a doctor applies a certain amount of pressure to these locations, they may hurt or be sensitive to the touch. Having pain in at least 11 of these sites was a clue that someone may have fibromyalgia.

Today, tender points are no longer needed to show if someone has fibromyalgia. Some people with fibromyalgia have tender points, while others with tender points don't have fibromyalgia.

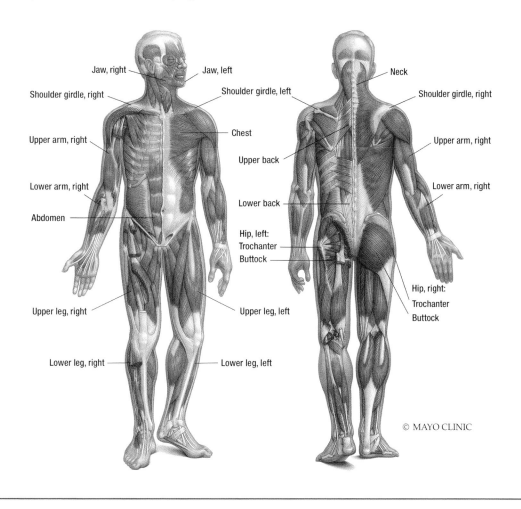

Jaw, right
Jaw, left
Neck
Shoulder girdle, right
Shoulder girdle, left
Shoulder girdle, right
Upper arm, right
Chest
Upper arm, right
Upper back
Lower arm, right
Lower arm, right
Abdomen
Lower back
Hip, left:
Trochanter
Buttock
Hip, right:
Trochanter
Buttock
Upper leg, right
Upper leg, left
Lower leg, right
Lower leg, left

© MAYO CLINIC

2. Pain in at least 11 of 18 tender point sites when pressure was applied. (Learn about tender points on the previous page.)

This list was a starting point for diagnosing fibromyalgia. But tender points were eventually removed from the criteria because there was no standard way to test and document them. Plus, some people with fibromyalgia didn't have tender points, while other people had tender points but didn't have fibromyalgia.

2010 guidelines

In 2010, the American College of Rheumatology revised its 1990 guidelines.

Under the updated guidelines, someone with fibromyalgia had to experience pain for at least three months with no other cause that could explain it. But tender points no longer had to be tested. Instead, the 2010 guidelines included a list of questions for a doctor to ask about an individual's pain.

For example, doctors asked their patients where they're feeling pain and how long their pain has been affecting them. A doctor would also inquire about an individual's medical history and try to find out if the person had symptoms that started in the joints, bones or skin within the last six months.

A doctor would also ask if someone was affected by fatigue, unrefreshing sleep, and problems with thinking or memory.

2011 changes to the guidelines

The 2010 guidelines offered a more complete picture of someone's symptoms, but it took a long time for a doctor to ask all of the necessary questions during an appointment and make a diagnosis.

This led to a change in the guidelines. People now could skip the interview process and fill out a questionnaire instead. The questionnaire let people list their symptoms without a doctor present. A doctor would then review the responses and final score to confirm if the person had fibromyalgia.

Alternative guidelines in 2013

In 2013, an alternative set of guidelines was released. These guidelines added more symptoms and included more areas of the body where someone might experience pain. Compared to the 2010/2011 guidelines, these newer guidelines added nine more areas where pain might be felt. (See how the lists compare on the next page.)

As with the 2010/2011 guidelines, people completed a survey to show which symptoms they had and how severe they were. A doctor would review the survey and indicate if the person had fibromyalgia.

Today's guidelines

The guidelines doctors use to diagnose fibromyalgia today were released in 2016.

Along with most of the aspects from the earlier guidelines, today's guidelines include some new components.

According to today's guidelines, someone with fibromyalgia must:

- Have a score that takes into consideration how widespread pain is and how severe symptoms are. This score is tallied based on someone's answers to questionnaires called a widespread pain index and a symptom severity scale.
- Have experienced pain in at least four of five parts of the body, not including the face and belly. These regions consist of the upper and lower left and right sides of the body and a fifth region that includes the neck, upper and lower back, chest, and belly.
- Have had symptoms of fibromyalgia, at about the same level, for at least three months.

FIBROMYALGIA: 2010/2011 VS 2013 GUIDELINES

Symptoms in the 2010/2011 guidelines	Symptoms in the 2013 guidelines
Fatigue	Pain
Waking up tired	Low energy
Thinking and memory issues	Stiffness
	Sleep problems
	Depression
	Memory problems
	Anxiety
	Tenderness to touch
	Balance problems
	Sensitivity to loud noises, bright lights, odors and cold

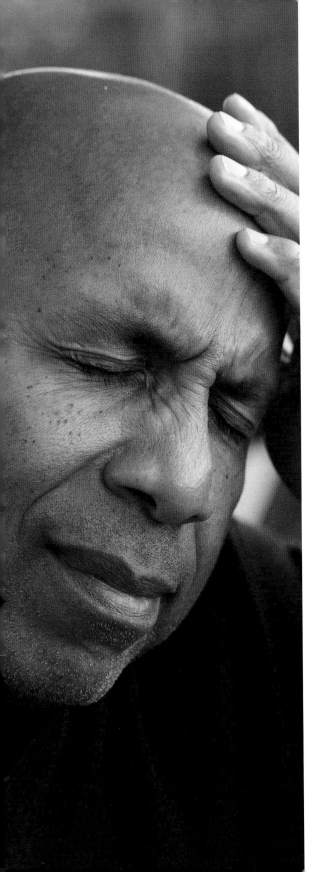

- Not have another disorder that can explain the pain. However, someone can have fibromyalgia even with another condition, whether it's related to fibromyalgia or not.

Some doctors still test tender points as part of their exam even though they aren't included in today's guidelines. But it's understood that while tender points may help a doctor determine if someone has fibromyalgia, tender points aren't always present in the condition.

OTHER SYMPTOMS

As you read earlier, fibromyalgia is thought to be linked to a process known as central sensitization (see page 47).

With central sensitization, communication between nerve sensors located all over your body and your brain gets turned up (amplified). This makes ordinary sensations feel more intense. A light touch may hurt, a quiet noise may sound much louder than it usually does and lights may seem unbearably bright.

Along with fibromyalgia, central sensitization is thought to cause several other disorders. This is why many people who have fibromyalgia often experience other symptoms and disorders in addition to fibromyalgia. It's also why you may have symptoms that seem unrelated to each other. In reality, they really may be related — through central sensitization.

Researchers have linked 25 symptoms to central sensitization. Here are the most common symptoms, many of which you may recognize in your experience with fibromyalgia. You got a glimpse of them earlier (see page 48); here's more on each one.

Fatigue

Fatigue is a defining symptom of central sensitization. It can come and go or always be present and doesn't go away after a night of sleep. It becomes chronic when you've experienced it for six months or more and no other medical condition can explain it.

Pain and tenderness

Half of the symptoms related to central sensitization are rooted in pain, whether it's muscle pain or joint pain. This pain doesn't seem to involve inflammation.

Numbness or tingling

If you're affected by central sensitization, you may feel numbness or tingling instead of or along with pain.

Headaches

Migraine and tension headaches are common symptoms of central sensitization. While tension headaches cause pain and pressure in the head, migraines can include other symptoms, too, such as nausea, vomiting, weakness, numbness, and extreme sensitivity to light and sound.

Brain fog

Thinking that feels faulty, memory problems or a short attention span all can happen with central sensitization. In relation to fibromyalgia, you may think of this symptom as "fibro fog."

Sleep problems

People experiencing central sensitization often have trouble sleeping. Some may sleep too much, while others either can't get enough sleep or wake unrefreshed. For those who snore a lot or are overweight, it's important to rule out sleep apnea first.

Dizziness and lightheadedness

Feeling dizzy and lightheaded may happen all the time, or just upon sitting or standing quickly.

Restless legs syndrome (RLS)

Central sensitization may affect the legs, causing a condition known as restless legs syndrome (RLS). People who have this condition describe crawling, pulling, throbbing, aching or itching sensations running through their legs, usually at night.

The only way to relieve the discomfort is to move the legs. RLS usually contributes to fatigue because it makes it difficult to sleep.

Temporomandibular joint (TMJ) dysfunction

Temporomandibular joint (TMJ) dysfunction involves pain in the joint and muscles around the jaw, with no sign of injury.

Irritable bowel syndrome (IBS)

IBS affects the large intestine (colon). Symptoms include cramps, belly pain, gas, diarrhea, bloating and constipation.

Interstitial cystitis

Interstitial cystitis causes pain and pressure in the bladder, frequent urination and pelvic pain. However, there's no sign of tissue damage or infection.

Weakness

A general sense of weakness may accompany central sensitization.

Chronic pelvic pain

Pelvic pain is pain felt below the bellybutton. It's different from menstrual cramping. In women who have central sensitization, chronic pelvic pain and menstrual pain often overlap, so doctors will typically rule out menstrual issues as the cause of chronic pelvic pain first.

Depression and anxiety

Depression and anxiety can accompany central sensitization. For many years, symptoms caused by central sensitization were believed to be all in the person's mind. Now, doctors understand that depression and anxiety can be caused by physical symptoms, but they can also lead to physical symptoms. The good news is that depression and anxiety are both very treatable.

Sensitivities

With central sensitization, the body may overreact to things in the environment. Food, light, sounds, medication and weather are all examples.

INSIDE THE DOCTOR'S OFFICE

Now that you know a little more about how doctors diagnose fibromyalgia, what should you do if you think you might have fibromyalgia but don't know for sure?

If you haven't been diagnosed with the condition, the first step is to talk to your doctor. The symptoms you're experiencing could be the sign of another medical condition, and that needs to be determined first.

If your symptoms aren't caused by another medical condition, your doctor can help lead you down the path of discovering whether you have fibromyalgia.

This may involve the help of a rheumatologist. A rheumatologist is a doctor specially trained to diagnose and treat conditions that affect the joints, muscles and bones. The key is to make sure that you get an accurate diagnosis of fibromyalgia from your doctor.

Here's a snapshot of the tests and steps that you may take to receive a diagnosis:

- **Medical history.** Your doctor will gather information about your medical history and any medications you're taking. You may also list disorders you've had in the past.
- **Screening.** Your doctor will likely ask you to complete the screening tests you learned about earlier in this chapter, including the widespread pain index and symptom severity scale surveys. These will help you indicate the symptoms you've had, how long you've had them and how they've been affecting you. You may also highlight areas on a diagram showing where you've experienced pain. Although you'll be responsible for filling out these surveys, your doctor will talk to you about your responses.
- **Blood tests.** Your doctor may order blood tests. Even though there's no specific test that can say if you have fibromyalgia, blood tests can uncover or rule out other conditions that may be causing your symptoms.

Keep in mind that even if the results of your tests point to something other than fibromyalgia, it's possible you could still have fibromyalgia. That's why it's critical to talk with your doctor and get a full exam to pinpoint exactly what's causing your symptoms.

Once you have a diagnosis, you can take steps toward managing its symptoms. You'll learn more about what this entails as you continue to read this book.

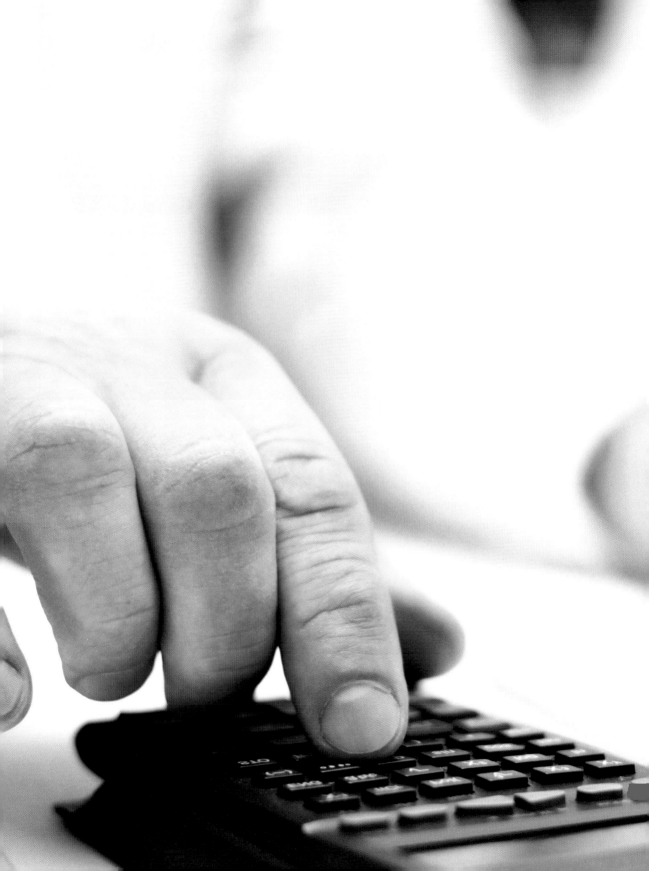

CHAPTER 6

The cost of fibromyalgia

So far, you've learned about what fibromyalgia is and what causes it. You've also gotten a glimpse into its effects through the personal stories that Gloria and Justus shared at the beginning of this book.

Given what you know now, you may wonder, *How much does fibromyalgia affect someone's life?* This chapter seeks to answer that question.

The cost of living with unmanaged fibromyalgia is high. It's high not just in terms of how much it can cost financially but also in how much it can cost physically, mentally and emotionally.

Use what you learn on the following pages as motivation to create a personalized, daily plan that will help you stave off many of the costs of fibromyalgia.

WHAT DOES FIBROMYALGIA COST?

What does fibromyalgia cost? It seems like this question should be easy to answer. All you need to do is figure out how much money is spent on health care visits, tests, medication and other treatments and add it up. Then you'll have a ballpark figure, right? Not exactly. Although some costs related to fibromyalgia can be measured in dollars and cents, the true, total cost can be much higher — and harder to put into numbers.

Fibromyalgia has been described as "iceberg" in nature. This means that fibromyalgia may seem harmless at first. After all, it doesn't get worse over time. It also isn't deadly. But its damage is hidden below the surface. On the outside, someone with fibromyalgia may look no different than anyone else. But inside the body, this disorder disrupts life in a number of ways.

Fibromyalgia can affect your job, your relationships and the activities you enjoy. Nothing in life is immune to its effects. You may have widespread pain for much of the day. You may be too tired to go to work or to even do simple household chores. You may find yourself struggling to remember even the most important items on your to-do list.

You may also be dealing with the effects of other conditions that are linked to fibromyalgia, which you learned about in Chapter 5. The effects of headaches, irritable bowel syndrome or depression, for example, can add to what you're already experiencing with fibromyalgia.

Fibromyalgia may feel daunting. Just the journey from diagnosis to treatment can test anyone's strength. Getting diagnosed is a process that many people who have fibromyalgia describe as long and stressful. It can take several years from the onset of symptoms, and it often means many visits to the doctor and several tests to rule out other causes for your symptoms.

Then, treatment enters the picture. Depending on your symptoms and how many you have, it may take several treatments — and several tries — to find what works for you.

But there's good news, too. With the right plan in place to manage your symptoms, you can overcome these challenges and even avoid much of what you'll read about in this chapter.

Financial hardship

If you have fibromyalgia, you may feel as if you spend more time in waiting rooms and with health care workers than you do anywhere and with anyone else.

Findings from research show why you may feel this way. Studies show that people with fibromyalgia may have anywhere from 10 to more than 20 visits to the doctor a year. When you break it down, that's one to two visits every month just for fibromyalgia. This also means more money out-of-pocket just for these visits. That doesn't include what it costs to get to and from appointments. Add testing and treatment to the mix, and fibromyalgia can cause a significant financial strain.

In one study, researchers analyzed the specific costs of fibromyalgia. They factored in the direct costs of dealing with fibromyalgia, including doctor visits, tests, medications and other treatment, and time spent in the hospital. Then they added indirect costs, such as disability, loss of work and wages,

"FIBRO FOG AFFECTS ANYWHERE FROM ONE-HALF TO NEARLY ALL PEOPLE WHO HAVE FIBROMYALGIA."

and costs related to basic daily needs, such as child care and housecleaning services.

When they added everything up, the researchers found that people who have severe fibromyalgia may spend $40,000 a year. More than $30,000 of this was linked to indirect costs of coping with the condition.

Workplace challenges

One of the mental challenges people with fibromyalgia face in the workplace is a symptom commonly referred to as "fibro fog." This term is used to describe the memory issues and short attention span associated with fibromyalgia. Although pain is the most common symptom of fibromyalgia, some people find that fibro fog can be even more disabling than the pain. It can affect how you interact with others and make it difficult to complete everyday tasks. Fibro fog affects anywhere from one-half to nearly all people who have fibromyalgia.

Pain, fatigue, poor sleep and depression that often come with fibromyalgia can also cause problems with recalling words or expressing thoughts. You may become more forgetful, your thinking may become disor-

ganized, and you may get distracted easily. These symptoms may make it difficult to adapt to a change in your environment, and your reaction time may slow.

For some people, the challenges of fibromyalgia lead them to stop working altogether. Of people who are diagnosed with fibromyalgia, 1 in 3 receives disability benefits, either short term or long term.

Those who continue to work may change jobs, work less or call in sick often, all due to their symptoms. Without work, it can be harder to pay bills, which adds stress to an already stressful situation. You'll learn more about disability in Chapter 19.

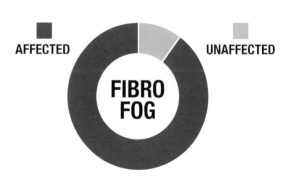

AFFECTED   **UNAFFECTED**

FIBRO FOG

Fibro fog affects anywhere from one-half to nearly all people who have fibromyalgia.

Loss of sleep

Nearly everyone with fibromyalgia has trouble sleeping. Falling asleep and getting enough deep sleep are typically the two biggest sleep issues. You may sleep lightly or not feel refreshed in the morning no matter how much sleep you get.

It's a vicious cycle. Pain reduces sleep quality, and not getting enough good sleep makes pain worse. Some research shows that poor sleep quality can make it more likely that you'll experience more of fibromyalgia's other effects, including anxiety and depression.

Poor sleep may also be linked to other effects of fibromyalgia, such as problems with memory and not being able to focus. In addition, many people who have fibromyalgia have trouble getting up in the morning because their sleep hasn't been restful or because they're in pain. You'll learn more about sleep issues in Chapter 16.

Fatigue

You may feel so tired that you have trouble doing even the simplest of things. One survey found that it often requires more time and more effort for someone with fibromyalgia to complete a task than it does for someone who doesn't have the condition. Survey participants indicated that fatigue was as much a part of their lives as the pain of fibromyalgia.

One survey responder put it this way: "You get 10 gallons of gas a day and you use them up in a certain way … when you are done, all of a sudden there you are standing at the kitchen sink and you just can't stand there another second. You can't cook anymore, you can't wash another dish. You just have to sit down."

You may find that you ration your energy, making sure you can do what needs to be done and putting everything else on the back burner. Cooking dinner may make the to-do list, but doing the laundry and watering the garden may have to wait.

In addition, you may find there are times when you have more energy, so you need to perform tasks during these hours — in the late morning to early afternoon, for example. Not being able to complete basic tasks can be upsetting, and you may come down hard on yourself for it.

Nine out of 10 people with fibromyalgia have trouble sleeping.

Moderation and pacing are important ways to keep fatigue from taking over your life. You'll learn how to use these techniques to your advantage in Chapter 14.

Physical deconditioning

If all you do is move from bed to chair to couch to bed, you can lose physical strength. This is known as physical deconditioning.

Deconditioning means that you can't move your body as well because you haven't been using your muscles. As you age, you can lose muscle mass. The same thing can happen with fibromyalgia. One study found that women who have fibromyalgia have only two-thirds of the muscle mass of women who don't have the condition.

You may feel as if your fibromyalgia is getting worse when it's actually your muscle strength that's decreasing. Getting out of bed or out of the bathtub can become difficult. Deconditioning decreases your quality of life and can threaten your independence. Deconditioning makes it harder to do things that you enjoy, such as hiking, gardening or traveling.

Physical deconditioning can also lead to more pain. When you don't use your muscles on a regular basis, less blood gets to your muscles. When you don't get enough blood to your muscles, you become more sensitive to pain. Deconditioning can also increase your risk of injury. It's another vicious cycle of fibromyalgia.

While some people who have fibromyalgia don't want to exercise because it hurts, nearly 4 out of 10 people who have fibromyalgia are actually afraid to move. This fear can also lead to the vicious cycle of deconditioning. Moving less leads to not being able to move as much, which in turn leads to more pain, more disability and more depression.

There is good news when it comes to physical deconditioning. You can address it and even prevent it by getting regular physical activity. Moving your muscles regularly can prevent muscle loss and pain related to it.

You already likely know that moving is good for you. But how can you do this when everything you do hurts, and you're exhausted all the time?

Research shows that low-impact exercises — walking, cycling and swimming are all examples — and strength training can help

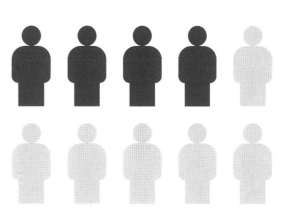

Nearly 4 out of 10 people who have fibromyalgia are actually afraid to move.

pain and improve muscle function. The key to making exercise help — and not hurt — is to start out slowly and work your way up gradually in terms of how hard and how long you exercise.

You'll learn how you can get physical activity back in your life, despite your pain and fatigue, in Chapter 13.

Strained relationships, feeling alone

Of people with fibromyalgia, half of them say they face struggles in their relationships.

More specifically, a survey from the National Fibromyalgia & Chronic Pain Association indicates that half the people with fibromyalgia feel that their condition has damaged their relationships with spouses or partners.

The survey also found that:
• More than 1 respondent in 4 felt that his or her spouse didn't understand fibromyalgia
• One respondent in 10 said that fibromyalgia helped lead to the breakup of a relationship
• One respondent in 4 said that his or her children thought the symptoms were being exaggerated

People may question your symptoms or even question your fibromyalgia altogether because they don't understand fibromyalgia, plus you may look healthy even though you're hurting. This misunderstanding can drive a wedge between you and the people you come in contact with — and even those closest to you. The stress of this situation may worsen your symptoms.

Relationships may be strained even further if you find yourself unable to make plans or commit to them because you're not sure of how you'll feel. Your children may feel resentful if you don't go to their games or play with them in the backyard. All the while, you wish you could spend more time with family and friends, but you don't because you hurt too much and are constantly tired.

Some people with fibromyalgia avoid seeing friends and family completely for fear they'll be criticized. If you do choose to (continued on page 76)

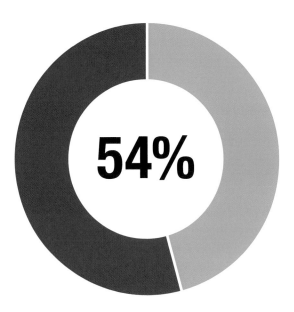

More than half the people with fibromyalgia say they face struggles in their relationships.

FIBROMYALGIA'S IMPACT ON MEN

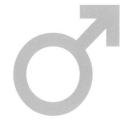

Fibromyalgia is often thought of as a disease that only affects women, but it also affects many men. In fact, more men are being diagnosed with fibromyalgia now than ever before. This is due mainly to recent changes in how fibromyalgia is diagnosed (see Chapter 5).

Under past guidelines, one man was diagnosed with fibromyalgia for every nine women who received the diagnosis. Newer criteria closes that gap. Now, one man is diagnosed with fibromyalgia for every two women who have the condition. Just as in women, the condition can be challenging to cope with — in some cases, maybe more so.

Some research suggests that men feel the same kind of pain that women feel in fibromyalgia. Other studies have found that men face more mental and emotional challenges and more physical limitations. Some researchers even suggest that men have a lower quality of life compared with women. One study participant indicated that fibromyalgia had completely changed his life and that he couldn't function at a level even close to what he could do before he was diagnosed with the condition. He said that fibromyalgia "has changed my entire life and the lives of my family."

Some men also feel that doctors don't take their symptoms seriously. In addition to widespread pain and feeling depressed and tired, they are also plagued with sleep issues and fibro fog.

Work problems can also cause concern. One survey found that many men with fibromyalgia missed considerable amounts of time at work, with some reporting that they'd missed as much as nine months of time on the job. Others said they lost their jobs because of their condition or had to file for disability because they could no longer work. Given the fact that men are often the breadwinners for their families, not being able to work can be costly not only financially but also in terms of self-esteem and self-worth.

HOW FIBROMYALGIA AFFECTS THE FAMILY

If you've recently been diagnosed with fibromyalgia, you're probably grappling with a mix of emotions and adjustments to your life.

Your family is also adapting to the changes that fibromyalgia has brought. Before you enlist your loved ones' support, it helps to think about how your condition may be affecting them. The more compassionate and understanding you can be toward your loved ones, the more the supportive they'll be for you.

Like you, your loved ones are in the process of wrapping their minds around the fact that you have a chronic condition. As they try to understand what that means for you and the family, they're likely wrestling with a host of feelings, including guilt, fear and anxiety.

Your loved ones may also be unsure about how fibromyalgia will affect your relationship with each of them. Family members may worry that your condition will restrict their day-to-day lives, forcing them to adapt to new routines or miss out on activities they've enjoyed in the past. They could also be struggling with feelings of helplessness in the face of your suffering or pain. These kinds of worries and emotions can cause stress in the family and put a strain on your relationships. This is especially true of your closest relationships, such as one with a spouse or partner.

You and your family may also experience tension over the way you each perceive your fibromyalgia symptoms. Because your pain and fatigue are invisible, your loved ones may not initially understand how severe your symptoms can be. At first, they may question whether your pain is truly that bad or why you need an extra nap. Such misunderstandings can be hurtful to you and cause conflict in the family.

It can help to remind yourself that your family members aren't inside your body. They have no way of knowing exactly what you're experiencing and will need time to fully grasp what fibromyalgia is like for you.

Just as their struggle to understand fibromyalgia can impact you, so can your struggles with fibromyalgia affect your family. Your loved ones may feel hurt or resentful when a flare in pain or fatigue prevents you from taking part in family activities or forces you to change plans. There may also be days when you're more irritable or short-tempered due to pain, fatigue and stress.

You don't have to ignore your feelings or put on a cheerful face all the time. But at the same time, it's important to try to focus on your abilities instead of your limitations. If you pay too much attention to the negative thoughts in your mind and get stuck in a glass-half-empty mentality, your relationships are more likely to suffer.

If there are times when you do take out your anger on your loved ones, ask for their understanding and let them know you're working on developing a more positive attitude.

In striving for a glass-half-full mindset, you'll be leading by example and setting a positive tone for your family.

With time, many families living with chronic disorders such as fibromyalgia come to accept the condition and work together to create a new normal. (Learn more in "Adjusting to a new normal" on page 227.)

These families see that it's possible to live well with fibromyalgia by working together as a team. They don't ignore the condition, but they also don't view it as something that needs to be the focus of or unduly interfere with family life. Rather than make fibromyalgia the center of their lives, these families find ways to continue engaging in many of the same activities as they did before, even if they have to make some changes to do so. Some families say that the experience of coping with a chronic condition has actually brought them closer together and strengthened their bond.

There's no question that fibromyalgia can challenge a family and put relationships to the test. But with kindness, patience, love and understanding, you can continue to share a warm, happy family life.

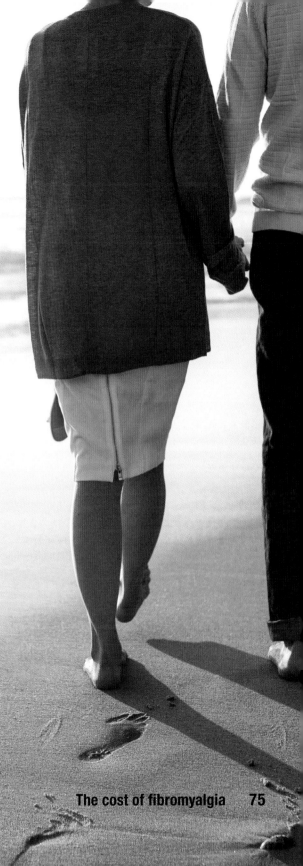

(continued from page 72)

share details about your fibromyalgia, you may get into arguments with well-intentioned family members or friends who are quick to offer advice on how to ease your symptoms.

There's also the shift in day-to-day responsibilities. Asking a spouse or partner to take on more household duties and child care can lead to feelings of resentment. Fibromyalgia also may affect your sex drive, creating more stress on a relationship. All of this can leave you feeling alone, as if no one believes you and you have no one to talk to.

It doesn't have to be this way. The support of family and friends is integral to helping you take back your life and live more fully with fibromyalgia.

The first step is knowing where to start and how to move forward together. In Chapter 18, you'll learn about ways you can repair strained or damaged relationships and get the support you need from your loved ones.

The toll on mental health

Based on what you've read so far in this book, it probably doesn't surprise you that fibromyalgia can cause feelings of depression, anger, fear or anxiety.

It's natural to have these feelings if you've gone months without a diagnosis or just learned you have fibromyalgia. In fact, adults with fibromyalgia are three times more likely to experience major depression than adults who don't have fibromyalgia.

You may feel anxious or depressed because you worry that your friends will abandon you because they don't understand your condition. You may worry that you'll lose your job. You may feel as if you've lost part of your identity, especially if you've had to change jobs or modify your daily tasks.

Unfortunately, many people don't talk about feelings of depression and anxiety with their health care team. They may worry that they'll be labeled as crazy. Or they become concerned that mentioning their depression or anxiety will distract their doctors from finding what's causing their pain and fatigue.

Research shows that depression can increase your risk of fibromyalgia — and at the same time, fibromyalgia makes depression more likely. If you're struggling with both fibromyalgia and depression, you may be even more exhausted. This can make it even harder to take steps that can help you feel better.

Even though you may be reluctant to do so, talk to your health care team about how you're feeling. Treating your depression and anxiety can help you better manage your fibromyalgia.

You'll learn more about steps you can take to lessen stress and improve your mood in Chapter 15.

Substance misuse

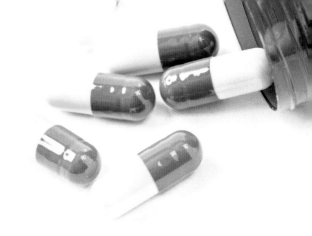

The use of opioids for chronic pain is a hot topic. Opioids are medications used to treat certain types of pain. But pain relief with opioids often comes at a high cost.

Opioids are highly addictive, and the United States has witnessed an alarming increase in drug overdoses as a result of opioids. How best to prescribe opioids and whether they should be used in the treatment of chronic pain is an ongoing discussion between doctors, government agencies and public officials.

Currently, no guidelines recommend using opioids for fibromyalgia pain. However, research indicates that 1 in 3 people who has fibromyalgia uses opioids.

Opioids carry many risks when they're used long term. According to some estimates, about 1 in 4 people who uses opioids for chronic pain misuses them. Drug overdoses are now the leading cause of death in adults under age 50 in the U.S., and opioids account for more than half of these deaths. In the span of a year, more than 42,000 people die of an overdose of these drugs. In addition, long-term opioid use may lead to even more pain, a condition known as hyperalgesia. You'll learn more about opioids in Chapter 7.

But opioids aren't the only problem. Mixing medications, taking medications with alcohol, and misusing alcohol or drugs are also concerns.

Research shows that alcohol misuse and chronic pain are connected. As many as 1 in 4 people with chronic pain misuses alcohol. And some research shows that between one-half and three-quarters of people who get treatment for an alcohol use disorder have moderate to severe pain. In one survey of individuals with widespread pain, the type of pain that happens in fibromyalgia, 1 in 5 respondents was a moderate to heavy drinker.

Mixing medications is also a concern for people dealing with chronic pain. In one study, 1 in 4 people who died of a drug overdose was taking opioids and gabapentin. You'll read more about gabapentin in Chapter 7.

As you can see, the cost of fibromyalgia is immeasurable. However, managing your symptoms can help you reclaim your life. In the chapters that follow, you'll learn about the steps you can take to start living your best life today.

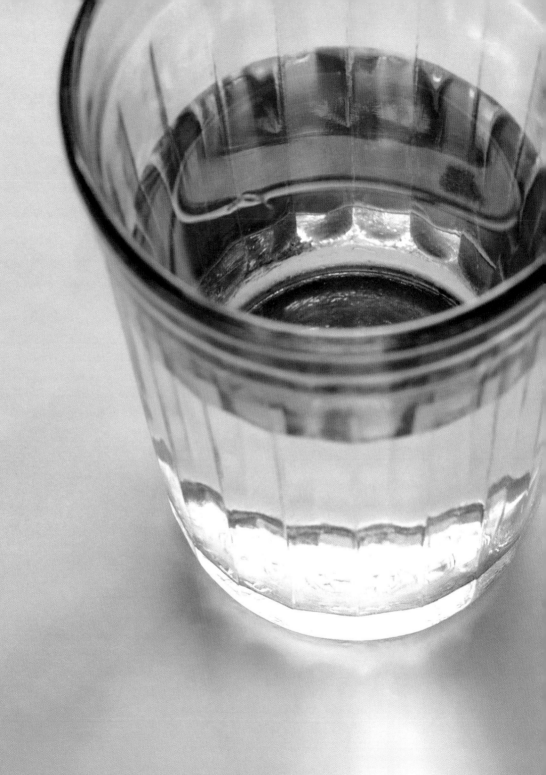

PART 2

Treating fibromyalgia

Now that you have a basic understanding of what fibromyalgia is, it's time to consider the best way to treat it.

When it comes to any kind of health issue, medication and integrative medicine are often the first two places people look for relief. For that reason, you'll learn about medications and integrative therapies that have been used to treat fibromyalgia. You'll discover that there are pros and cons to both approaches. You'll also get an inside look at special programs and centers that focus on

helping people manage fibromyalgia and other pain-related conditions.

As you read through this part of the book, keep in mind that fibromyalgia has no cure yet. This is not a condition that is likely to disappear. And at this point, it's not a condition that any medication can "fix." With that said, there are therapies and techniques that can help you manage your symptoms, no matter what they are.

The next few chapters will help set the stage for a personalized, effective plan that you can use every day to manage your symptoms and, more importantly, enjoy your life.

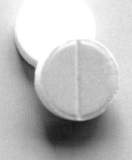

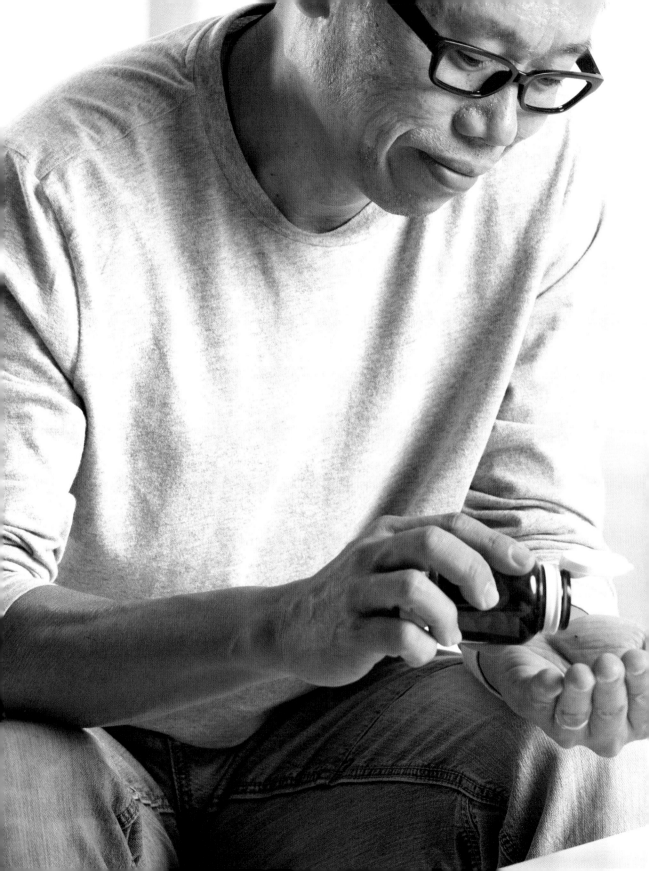

CHAPTER 7

Medications

Fibromyalgia is a pain disorder. That means pain is the main symptom of this condition. With this in mind, think of other times when you've felt pain. Maybe you sprained an ankle, for example. In this case, it makes sense to take a pain reliever to ease your pain while your injury heals. But fibromyalgia is different. It's not acute pain like a sprained ankle. Instead, the pain is chronic, meaning that it lasts over a long period of time.

Either way — whether you've sprained your ankle or you have fibromyalgia — you have pain. So in both cases, it's best to rely on medication to feel better, right? In reality, the answer to this question isn't that simple.

The fact is, pain medication is just one part of treatment for fibromyalgia. Other types of medication can help address other symptoms of the condition. But what to use, how

to use it, and the risks and benefits vary from person to person.

No one medication can relieve all of your fibromyalgia symptoms all of the time. And in many cases, medication may not help at all or may even make you feel worse.

In this chapter, you'll learn about medications that have been approved to help treat fibromyalgia. You'll learn about how they work, and their pros and cons.

PAIN MEDICATIONS 101

Now that you have an understanding about what fibromyalgia is and isn't, let's focus on its main symptom: pain.

The pain of fibromyalgia never seems to go away, although how much you hurt may vary from day to day. The condition is chronic, which means it lasts longer than three months. This is different from acute pain that's part of everyday life, from something as minor as a paper cut to something as serious as surgery or a broken bone. Acute pain usually stems from an obvious cause, which also makes it different from the pain of fibromyalgia.

Many types of medications are used to treat acute pain. They relieve the pain until what caused it has healed. In time, acute pain goes away. Chronic pain, on the other hand, doesn't always have an obvious cause and doesn't go away.

All of these differences between acute pain and the chronic pain of fibromyalgia signal a need to take a closer look at pain medications, how they're used, and which, if any, you should consider using to help treat your fibromyalgia symptoms. Not all pain medications are created equal, and not all pain medications should be used to relieve every type of pain.

Several different types of pain medications are available, and medications used to treat other conditions are sometimes prescribed to treat fibromyalgia, too. This chapter of-

fers insight into the main medications used to treat fibromyalgia and what's known about them.

TREATMENT OPTIONS

Unlike many other conditions, fibromyalgia has no cure. The focus of fibromyalgia treatment is to relieve symptoms rather than cure the condition. And as far as medications are concerned, no single drug can relieve all of its symptoms.

With this said, three medications have been approved by the Food and Drug Administration (FDA) to treat fibromyalgia:
- Pregabalin (Lyrica)
- Duloxetine (Cymbalta)
- Milnacipran (Savella)

You'll learn how these drugs work, as well as their risks and benefits, starting on the next page. Your doctor may choose to use these approved drugs or other drugs described as "off-label." Off-label drugs are not approved by the FDA for fibromyalgia, but your doctor may suggest trying them to help relieve your symptoms. If some symptoms are more severe than others, this may help guide your doctor toward suggesting one medication over another. You'll learn more about all of these drugs as you continue to read this chapter.

With any medication you try, it's important to be patient and give it time to work. You may not notice an improvement in your symptoms for several weeks.

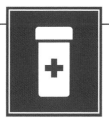

TRICYCLIC ANTIDEPRESSANTS

Antidepressants affect chemicals in the brain that are responsible for helping to regulate and improve mood and reduce pain. Tricyclic antidepressants are one of the two main types of antidepressants used to treat fibromyalgia, and they're often one of the first medications suggested for people who have fibromyalgia. They're used to help ease pain and fatigue and may improve sleep. The other type of antidepressant often used to treat fibromyalgia is on the next page.

Name: Amitriptyline, others

How effective are they? Research shows that antidepressants can help ease symptoms of fibromyalgia. However, their effectiveness — how much they help — may decrease over time.

Tricyclic antidepressants are widely available and at a lower cost than some of the other medications used to treat fibromyalgia. If you respond to these medications, you may see improvement in many signs and symptoms, including fatigue, pain, sleep problems, and bowel and bladder issues.

Potential side effects: Dry mouth, weight gain, fluid retention, constipation, trouble concentrating, feeling "drugged."

Who shouldn't take them: People who take antidepressants called monoamine oxidase inhibitors (MAOIs) and people who've had a recent heart attack or have certain other heart conditions.

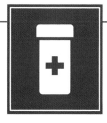

SEROTONIN AND NOREPINEPHRINE REUPTAKE INHIBITORS (SNRIS)

You read about tricyclic antidepressants on the previous page. The other type of antidepressant often used to treat fibromyalgia symptoms is serotonin and nor-epinephrine reuptake inhibitors (SNRIs), also known as dual reuptake inhibitors. Like tricyclic antidepressants, SNRIs affect chemicals in the brain that are responsible for helping to regulate and improve mood and reduce pain.

Names: Duloxetine (Cymbalta), milnacipran (Savella)

How effective are they? SNRIs tend to be the most effective antidepressants for treating many symptoms at once. Which medication you take depends on your symptoms. Duloxetine may be used to help relieve pain and may help with severe fatigue and depression. Milnacipran may be used if you also have severe fatigue or memory issues.

Duloxetine has been shown to help relieve fibromyalgia pain. Some people with and without depression have found this medication helpful for fibromyalgia. It may also help reduce mental fatigue. Research shows that milnacipran can help lessen pain and improve physical function.

Potential side effects: Nausea, feelings of a fast-beating, fluttering or pounding heart even at rest, headache, constipation, fatigue, high blood pressure, problems sleeping, thoughts of suicide.

Who shouldn't take them: People who take an MAOI, have certain forms of the eye disease glaucoma, have a history of alcohol abuse, or have liver or kidney damage.

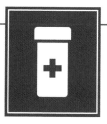

MUSCLE RELAXERS

A muscle relaxer may be a first treatment if you have mild to moderate fibromyalgia symptoms. Muscle relaxers are sometimes used to help promote sleep. They're similar to tricyclic antidepressants in their chemical structure and are thought to help symptoms in a similar way.

Name: Cyclobenzaprine (Amrix)

How effective are they? A small research trial found that a low dose of cyclobenzaprine helps improve sleep and may help reduce pain and improve symptoms of fatigue and depression. However, cyclobenzaprine isn't considered a depression treatment.

Muscle relaxers are widely available. They often also cost less than some of the other medications used to treat fibromyalgia. They may improve several signs and symptoms, including fatigue, pain, sleep problems, and bowel and bladder issues.

Potential side effects: Dry mouth, weight gain, fluid retention, constipation, trouble concentrating, feeling "drugged."

Who shouldn't take them: People taking MAOIs or who have recently stopped taking them, people who have allergies to any of the drug's ingredients, people who have hyperthyroidism, and people who have had a recent heart attack or who have heart problems such as heart rhythm disturbances (arrhythmias) or congestive heart failure.

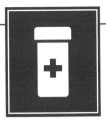

ANTI-SEIZURE MEDICATIONS

Drugs used to treat seizure conditions are sometimes used to treat chronic pain. Research shows that two anti-seizure drugs — pregabalin and gabapentin — may help with fibromyalgia pain by affecting the body's pain pathways.

Names: Pregabalin (Lyrica), gabapentin (Gralise, Horizant, Neurontin)

How they work: They're thought to block the excessive firing of certain nerve cells (neurons) in the brain that are responsible for feelings of pain.

How effective are they? If amitriptyline hasn't worked for you, or if you have severe sleep issues as well as pain, pregabalin may be an option. If you find that pregabalin is too expensive, your doctor may recommend gabapentin instead. Pregabalin has been shown to reduce fibromyalgia pain for some people. In some studies, it's also been shown to improve sleep, feelings of tiredness and quality of life. Not all research shows these benefits.

Compared with pregabalin, gabapentin doesn't have as much evidence to support its use in treating fibromyalgia. The limited research that's been done suggests that gabapentin may help relieve pain. However, newer research reports that there's potential for misuse in people who use gabapentin. Most often, this misuse happens with people who have used opioids or a class of drugs called benzodiazepines.

Potential side effects: Drowsiness, weight gain, dizziness, dry mouth, swelling of the limbs.

Who shouldn't take them: Anyone who has had a reaction to these medications or any of their ingredients.

WHEN ONE DRUG ISN'T EFFECTIVE

Fibromyalgia's web of symptoms is complex. This may explain why most people take more than one medication to treat their symptoms. They're not necessarily taking full doses of all of their medications, though. Some research shows that the majority never take full doses of their medications. At the one-year mark, only about 1 in 5 people is still taking medication at all.

If you're taking the maximum dosage of a single medication but you aren't getting relief from your symptoms, it may be time for a change.

Although research doesn't seem to show that combining drugs is helpful, your doctor may suggest adding other medications to your plan. If you and your doctor feel that your daily plan for managing your symptoms is in good shape but you're still not getting enough relief from your symptoms, your doctor may suggest the following alternative medications.

Alternative medications for symptoms

These medications are limited in terms of how much they can help, but you and your doctor may decide they're worth trying. Here's information on each type of medication and how it may help.

Analgesics Analgesics, which include acetaminophen (Tylenol, others) and a weak opioid called tramadol (Ultram, Conzip),

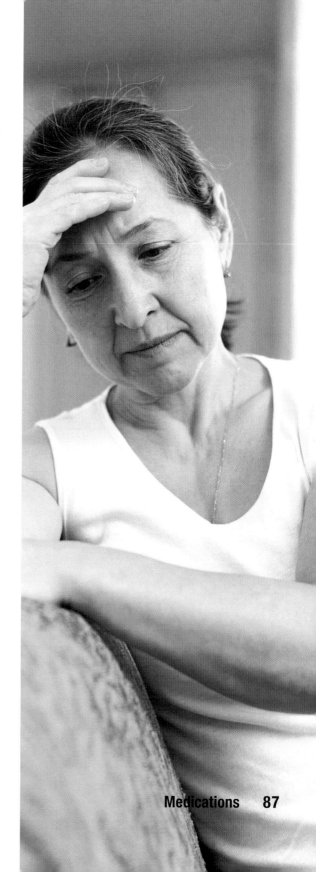

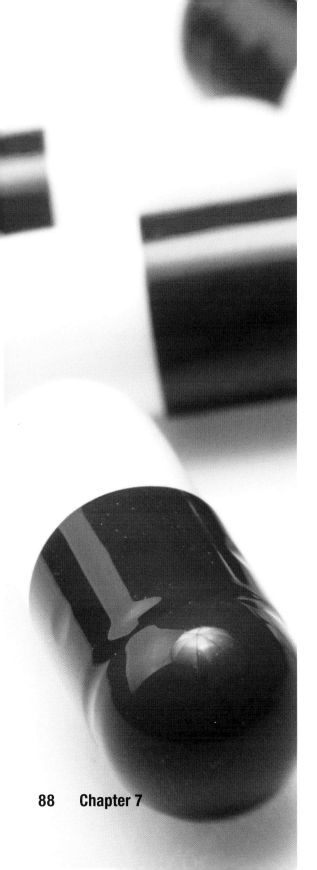

may be used together to address fibromyalgia flare-ups and temporarily relieve pain. Caution is needed here, however, because tramadol is an opioid. (See "The problem with opioids" on page 89.)

Selective serotonin reuptake inhibitors (SSRIs) Research around the use of the antidepressants SSRIs in treating fibromyalgia is mixed. Most studies that have been done have been of low quality.

But some evidence suggests that older SSRIs, such as fluoxetine (Prozac, Sarafem, Selfemra), sertraline (Zoloft) and paroxetine (Brisdelle, Paxil, Pexeva), taken in higher doses may be better for relieving pain than newer SSRIs, such as citalopram (Celexa), escitalopram (Lexapro), and desvenlafaxine (Khedezla, Pristiq). These drugs may cause nausea, sexual dysfunction, weight gain and trouble sleeping.

Options beyond medications

You may find that taking only one medication isn't helping you. If you're reluctant to add more medications to the mix, this may be a good time to review your entire plan for managing your symptoms and find non-drug therapies you can use instead.

USING OPIOIDS TO TREAT FIBROMYALGIA

In the middle of the 20th century, a new model for managing pain emerged: interdisciplinary pain rehabilitation. You'll learn about this concept in Chapter 10. Although this approach is seen as an effective way to manage fibromyalgia symptoms today, it took time for these programs to take off.

In the meantime, an increasing focus on addressing pain emerged in the 1990s. The American Pain Society's campaign "Pain: the 5th Vital Sign" stressed the importance of evaluating pain and treating it. There was also a shift away from earlier fears of opioids and addiction risks. Instead, doctors were in favor of treating and relieving pain and improving patient satisfaction.

All of this created a perfect storm for increasing the use of opioid medications. The opioid oxycodone (OxyContin) went from 670,000 prescriptions written in 1997 to about 6.2 million prescriptions in 2002.

The problem with opioids

More than half the people with fibromyalgia take some form of opioid as part of their treatment.

This is concerning for a number of reasons:
- Over time, you may develop a tolerance to the drug. This means that your body gets used to the dose you're taking. This leads to a need to increase your dose over and over again to achieve the same level of pain relief. This may mean taking up to 10 times the original dose.
- Some people who take opioids for fibromyalgia develop a condition called hy-peralgesia. This means that your body feels pain more, the exact opposite of what taking a pain medication is meant to achieve. Pain medication is supposed to relieve pain, not cause more of it. Hyperalgesia may lead you to take higher doses of opioids than you should.
- Abruptly stopping opioids can lead to withdrawal symptoms. Withdrawal symptoms vary in terms of how severe they are. The medication you're taking, how much of it you're taking and how long you've been taking it all factor in to the withdrawal symptoms you may experience. Common signs and symptoms of withdrawal include chills, sleep problems, diarrhea, nausea, vomiting and muscle aches. Symptoms of withdrawal can last up to two weeks. Gradually reducing how much medication you're taking is important for avoiding symptoms of withdrawal.

Risk of addiction Another risk related to taking opioids for chronic pain is the risk of addiction. Estimates vary, but a review of people being treated for chronic pain at pain clinics found that an average of 1 in 10 was addicted to opioids.

Addiction is a risk even if you take an opioid as prescribed. It's a risk even if you don't have a history of substance abuse or mental illness, both of which can make addiction more likely. Addiction is more common if you take opioids for long periods of time, but you're still at risk of becoming addicted to opioids even if you take them only for a short time.

MEDICATIONS AT A GLANCE

Medication and symptoms it may help	Pain	Fatigue	Sleep problems	Depression	Cognitive problems
Amitriptyline	✔	✔	✔		
Cyclobenzaprine	✔		✔		
Duloxetine	✔		✔	✔	
Milnacipran	✔	✔			✔
Pregabalin	✔		✔		
Tramadol	✔				

Based on Skaer TL. Current issues regarding the care of the fibromyalgia patient. *Fibromyalgia: Open Access.* 2017;2:120. Goldenberg DL, et al. Initial treatment of fibromyalgia in adults. *http://www.uptodate.com/contents/search.*

It's important to understand the difference between addiction and dependence. It's possible to become dependent on a medication but not addicted to it.

Dependence on a pain medication is common and involves two specific parts of the brain, the thalamus and the brainstem. When you're dependent and you stop taking medication, you experience withdrawal symptoms. However, with dependence, there isn't a compulsive need to use the medication. That is addiction.

Addiction to a medication involves the brain's reward pathway. You may find yourself unable to stop using the drug even though it's having a negative impact on your life, such as causing problems with work, friends or family.

POSSIBLE SIDE EFFECTS OF OPIOID USE

Short-term use	Long-term use
Bladder problems	Misuse and addiction
Irregular heartbeat	Tolerance that leads to taking higher and higher doses
Constipation	Problems with hormones
Nausea	Feeling pain more than you used to
Vomiting	
Impaired thinking, including a slower reaction time	
Muscle spasms	
Stiff muscles	
Dizziness	
Itchy skin	
Fever	
Breathing problems	
Sleepiness or problems sleeping	
Sexual dysfunction	

WHAT ABOUT MARIJUANA?

Many people who have fibromyalgia try medication after medication, seeking relief from their symptoms. You may be able to relate to this. In turn, if nothing else has seemed to help, you may wonder if marijuana might be worth trying.

Medical marijuana has been approved for use in some states for some conditions. However, the Food and Drug Administration (FDA) has not approved marijuana for use in treating fibromyalgia.

Recent research shows that the chemicals in marijuana may work not by relieving pain but by helping pain feel less unpleasant and more tolerable. But how well these chemicals work is still up for debate. Some studies suggest that both natural and man-made forms of the compounds in marijuana help with pain and improve sleep. But other research suggests that marijuana doesn't have much of an effect on fibromyalgia pain. One very small study showed that smoking marijuana may slightly help people with fibromyalgia in terms of their mental and emotional health, but the study was too small for a recommendation to be made for its use. Safety concerns and side effects are two more reasons that marijuana is not recommended for treating pain.

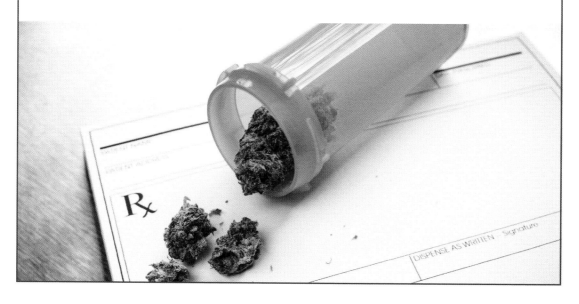

Opioids: What should you do?

Despite all of the risks involved with taking opioids, there are certain instances in which they can be beneficial. Opioids are often used for a short period to treat acute pain, such as pain after surgery.

But opioids *aren't* recommended for the treatment of chronic pain, such as the pain of fibromyalgia.

If you're taking an opioid to treat your fibromyalgia pain and you want to stop taking it for any reason, dose tapering can help. In fact, you may find that your pain actually *improves* after your body adjusts to not taking the medication. Gradually taper your dose with help from your doctor.

TO MEDICATE … OR NOT

In the absence of a treatment that can completely relieve fibromyalgia symptoms, deciding whether to take medications is one that's best made by carefully weighing the pros and cons with your health care team.

Medication may help dial down the pain you're experiencing, boost your mood or reduce your fatigue. You may find it easier to sleep at night.

But taking medication may also cause side effects. You'll need to decide if the benefits of taking medication outweigh the problems they may cause. In some cases, the side effects may be severe enough to make you quit taking the medication. And over time, some medications may not work as well.

Drug therapy is rarely recommended as the only treatment for fibromyalgia's symptoms. It may help, but it should be used as only one part of a comprehensive plan. Research bears this out: In one analysis, all of the management strategies people with fibromyalgia found to be the most effective were nondrug therapies.

One final caveat: If you find your medication isn't working or seems to have lost effectiveness, it's best not to take it. This helps reduce your risk of side effects and interactions with other medications. But don't quit it cold turkey. Talk to your doctor about other treatment options, including different medications and other nondrug choices you can make.

The chapters that follow will help you explore nondrug options for managing your fibromyalgia and living your best life even with this condition.

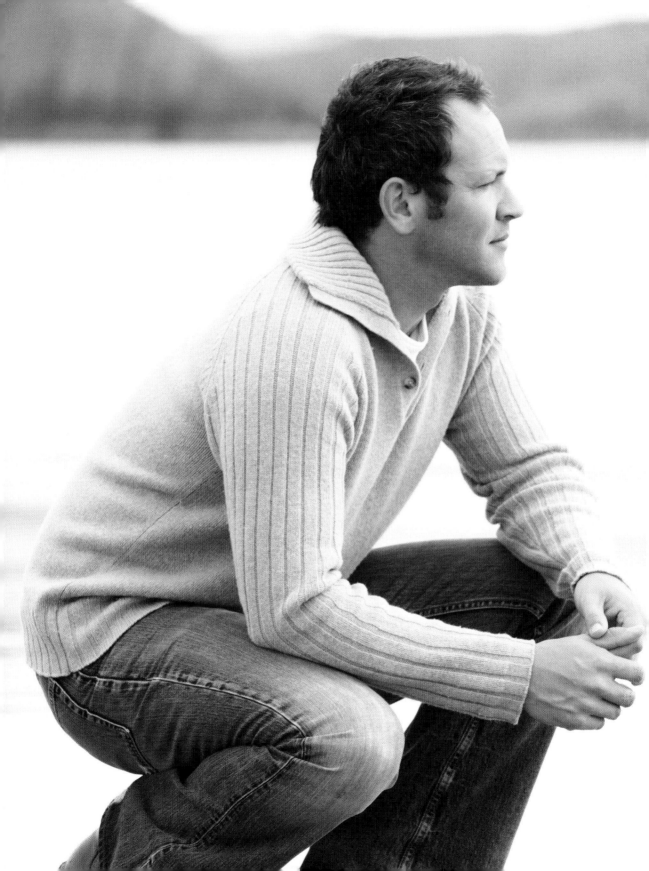

CHAPTER 8

Cognitive behavioral therapy

What you think, how you feel and what you do about fibromyalgia can have a powerful effect on your life — for the better.

In this chapter, you'll learn about cognitive behavioral therapy. At its core, cognitive behavioral therapy helps you replace negative or inaccurate thoughts with thoughts that are more positive and realistic. You then use your thoughts and feelings to change your behavior. The goal of cognitive behavioral therapy is to help you recognize that fibromyalgia is something you can manage. When you feel confident about your ability to manage your symptoms, your entire life can improve.

Cognitive behavioral therapy is the most effective way to manage fibromyalgia. It's the basis for the techniques featured in the chapters that follow in this book.

CHANGING YOUR APPROACH TO FIBROMYALGIA

What if you could:
- Manage your pain and other symptoms, rather than having them run your life, day in and day out
- Learn techniques that can help you cope with pain and other symptoms more effectively than you are now
- Change how you think and feel about your pain and other symptoms so that they don't affect you as much
- Feel confident about managing your symptoms

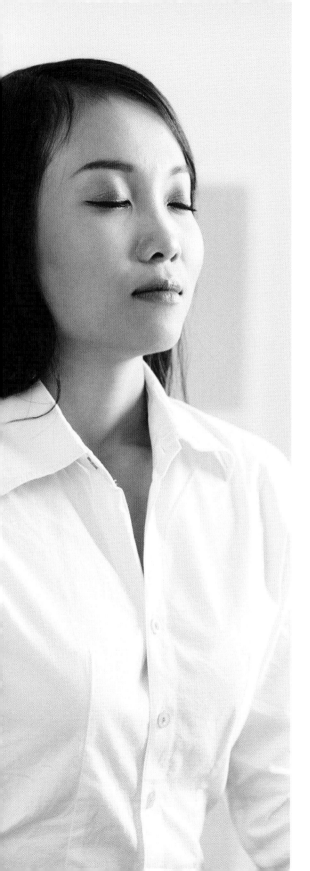

- Anticipate problems before they happen and solve them before they have a chance to take hold of your life
- Return to a life that you enjoy

You can do all of this by changing what you think, feel and do. That's the basis of cognitive behavioral therapy.

In this chapter, you'll learn how you can apply cognitive behavioral therapy to fibromyalgia. In the chapters that follow, you'll learn more about how to put it into practice.

CHANGING YOUR THOUGHTS, BEHAVIORS AND FEELINGS

Cognitive behavioral therapy helps you cope with fibromyalgia by changing how you think about it and respond to it. It's been used to effectively treat a variety of pain syndromes. It also teaches ways to cope with stressful life situations.

Cognitive behavioral therapy teaches you to challenge negative thoughts and adopt more realistic ways of thinking. In turn, you learn to believe in your ability to manage fibromyalgia and change the way you think about your pain — and change how it makes you feel.

Here's a step-by-step look at how cognitive behavioral therapy works:

1. Identify troubling situations or conditions in your life. These are the situations that cause you to feel stressed. Maybe you

COGNITIVE BEHAVIORAL THERAPY: BEFORE AND AFTER

The situation: You get criticism from a co-worker.

Without cognitive behavioral skills:

What you think: I can't do anything right or No one likes me.
How you feel: Sad, anxious, stressed; your muscles tense up.
Actions you take: You avoid your manager or call in sick to work.
Results: You think, *I'm behind in my work, I'll never catch up* or *I'm going to get fired. Why bother going to work?*

This situation shows how hard it can be to control thoughts that lead to distress. Worry can help you work through problems, but in many cases, it only leads you to spend more time thinking about your problems instead of how to solve them. The longer you think about your problems, the worse you tend to feel.

With cognitive behavioral skills:

What you think: I try to do my best at work. Most of the feedback I get is positive.
How you feel: You feel less sad and anxious and have less tension.
Actions you take: Make an appointment to talk to your manager about your performance. You continue going to work.
Results: You feel that you're keeping up with work, and you feel more aware of positive feedback from others. This helps you feel more confident.

In this situation, negative thoughts and worries don't have a chance to take hold because you took time to look at how and what you're thinking. This helps you reframe the criticism you got from your co-worker. Instead of jumping to negative thoughts and worry, you realized that there's a more realistic and positive way to look at the criticism you received.

"THESE STEPS ARE BASED ON THE IDEA THAT YOUR THOUGHTS CAN EITHER HELP YOU OR HURT YOU."

worry that you won't be able to work again or that you won't be as good a friend, spouse or parent.

2. Become aware of what you think, how you feel and what you believe about these problems. With this step, you learn to recognize when you're having negative thoughts.

3. Identify thoughts that are negative or inaccurate. Are you really a terrible parent, for example, or are you being too hard on yourself because you feel less able to play with your kids like you did before?

4. Replace negative thoughts with thoughts that are more realistic and accurate. Instead of telling yourself, *This pain will never get better,* for example, you may tell yourself, *I can handle this. I have done it before, and I can do it again.*

These four steps help you reshape your thoughts and feelings. The steps are based on the idea that your thoughts can either help you or hurt you. That's the *cognitive* part of cognitive behavioral therapy.

You can tell yourself, *I can't do that* or *That will never work.* Or, you can exchange those

thoughts for more realistic and positive ones, such as, *I can do this.*

Cognitive behavioral therapy can help you cope with fibromyalgia in a more realistic way. When you face a challenge or obstacle, taking this approach can help you feel less distressed. The strategies you learn are designed to help you feel encouraged, happy, calm, content and confident about your ability to manage your symptoms and the challenges they bring to your life.

The *behavioral* part of cognitive behavioral therapy addresses the active part of living with fibromyalgia. It includes setting goals, action planning, engaging with people, attending activities, and stretching and physical movement. Put simply, it means truly living your life and not letting fibromyalgia or its symptoms hold you back.

Behavioral strategies include getting more physical activity and learning to pace yourself so that you're not doing too much on your good days but are still staying active, even on your bad days. Other behavioral strategies include steps you can take to sleep better and relaxation techniques such as deep breathing or mindfulness meditation to help you relax.

WHAT SKILLS WILL YOU LEARN?

Cognitive behavioral therapy teaches skills aimed at helping you manage your pain and other symptoms. You've started to learn about some of these skills; you'll learn about others in the chapters that follow.

- Pacing and time management
- Progressive muscle relaxation, which is when you relax all of the muscles in your body in a sequence, one muscle group at a time
- Guided imagery, which is when you form mental images of places or situations you find relaxing
- Strategies to help you sleep better
- How to schedule activities that you enjoy
- Ways to reframe your thoughts so that they're more positive and realistic
- Memory and thinking skills
- How to talk to your health care team
- Goal setting
- Self-monitoring

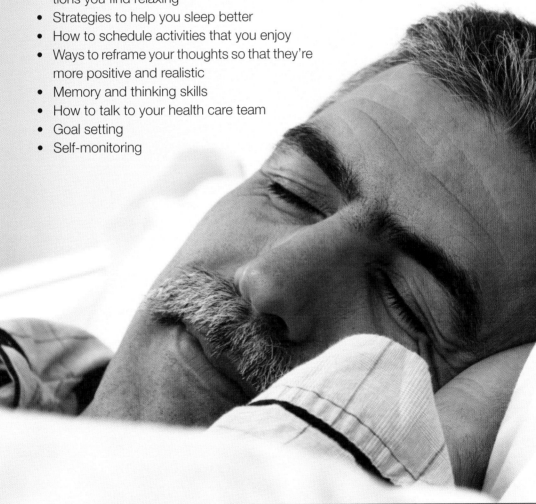

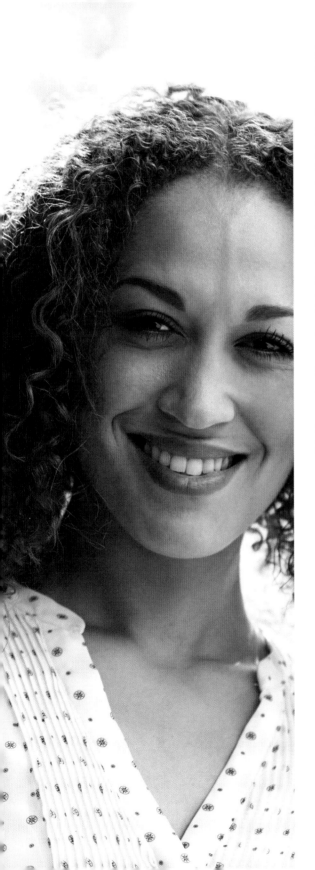

How well does cognitive behavioral therapy work?

Cognitive behavioral therapy has been used for many years to help treat a variety of physical challenges, from losing weight to managing headaches. In 1998, researchers wondered whether cognitive behavioral therapy could help treat fibromyalgia, too. An early study indicated that combining education, meditation and movement therapy could help people with fibromyalgia reduce their pain, function better and improve their mood. These tenets of cognitive behavioral therapy are all used today to treat fibromyalgia.

Since then, hundreds of studies have found that the therapy can treat a range of pain syndromes, including fibromyalgia. Today, it's the most commonly accepted way to help people cope with pain.

Studies suggest that programs using cognitive behavioral therapy to teach people how to manage pain are effective because cognitive behavioral therapy treats the physical side of pain and addresses how people think and feel about it. Cognitive behavioral therapy supports the idea that healthy behaviors can help with managing symptoms.

It also reinforces the idea of refocusing attention away from pain and other symptoms. Paying attention to something other than pain can make pain feel less intense. When people distract themselves from pain, brain images show less activity in the part of the brain that deals with pain.

TOP 5 TECHNIQUES

These five cognitive behavioral therapy techniques in particular are helpful in coping with fibromyalgia. That's why you're reading about them in this book:

- Relaxation techniques
- Pacing and regular exercise
- Social support
- Diverting attention away from pain and other symptoms
- Trying new coping strategies for pain, such as replacing negative responses to pain and other symptoms with more realistic responses

In one study, after several weeks of using these strategies, people with fibromyalgia felt better equipped to manage their pain.

This technique has been shown to relieve pain as well as — and in some cases, even better than — pain-relieving medications.

Even simply thinking about pain differently can help. Instead of telling yourself, *This pain is never going to get better,* you may tell yourself, *I can handle this pain.*

Other examples of cognitive behavioral therapy techniques — such as guided imagery, meditation and mindfulness-based stress reduction, which teaches ways to manage and reframe thoughts that are worrisome or negative — can lessen the effect that symptoms have on your life.

In addition to pain, cognitive behavioral therapy can be helpful in treating anxiety and depression, both of which are common with fibromyalgia. Some researchers suggest that cognitive behavioral therapy is so effective for anxiety and depression it should be the treatment of choice.

People of all ages coping with a chronic pain condition can benefit from cognitive behavioral therapy. It's especially helpful when it's combined with other types of treatment, such as aerobic exercise, strength training, a healthy diet and medication if needed.

With cognitive behavioral therapy, you're in the driver's seat. You can choose not to let pain run your life, and you have the power to deal with your pain in ways that enable you to live life more fully — and enjoy it.

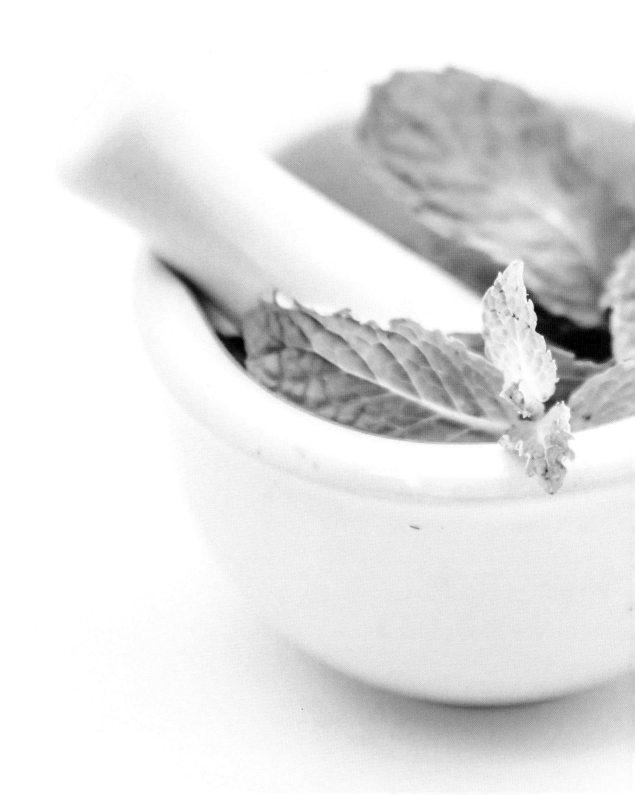

CHAPTER 9

Integrative medicine

Integrative medicine is the practice of using conventional medicine along with complementary treatments that have been shown to help manage or treat a condition. For example, if you have high blood pressure, you may take medication but also practice deep breathing to bring your blood pressure down to a healthy level. Integrative medicine doesn't replace conventional medicine. Instead, it's used to *complement* conventional medicine. That's why you may hear it called complementary medicine.

In Chapter 4, you learned about central sensitization. This is the idea that in fibromyalgia, the nervous system is "turned up" or on high alert. Therapies in this chapter help "turn down" the messages about pain and other symptoms that get to the brain. In turn, you can reduce the signs and symptoms you're feeling, including pain.

Integrative medicine has become more and more popular in the last 20 years, and interest in it continues to grow. This is especially true for people who don't feel as though they're getting the help they need from conventional medicine. This chapter offers the latest information on integrative therapies that are commonly used for fibromyalgia, including how effective they are. The information in this chapter will help you on your journey toward developing a plan for managing your symptoms.

WHAT IS INTEGRATIVE MEDICINE?

You may recognize integrative medicine as "alternative medicine" or "complementary and alternative medicine." Today, these practices and therapies are known as integrative medicine because doctors are using them along with conventional medicine.

Here are several integrative therapies that have been used to treat fibromyalgia. By and large, they focus mostly on managing pain and stress.

Relaxation exercises

As you'll learn later in this book (see page 182), relaxation exercises are an important part of managing fibromyalgia symptoms. They're also a type of integrative medicine. Here are several types of relaxation exercises and how they work. Learn how to do some of these exercises on page 254.

These exercises are all simple to try. You don't need special equipment, and you can use them anytime, anywhere.

Guided imagery Close your eyes and use all of your senses to imagine a scene that brings about feelings of peace. Use all of your senses to experience the location as fully as you can. This is the basis of guided imagery.

Guided imagery relies on focus and mindfulness. You use the power of your imagination to take you to places you find relaxing. This can help you feel more at ease and feel less pain.

Research has shown that guided imagery can help relieve symptoms of fibromyalgia. For example, people who've found it helpful have said that they felt less stress, fatigue, pain and depression.

Meditation Meditation involves calmly focusing on the present moment. It can help quiet your mind and relax your muscles.

Most types of meditation require four elements: a quiet place, a specific posture, focused attention and an open mind.

Deep breathing Breathing is likely something that you don't think much about. Your chest rises and falls, and that's likely all the thought you give to it.

Deep breathing is different. When you breathe normally, your chest rises and falls. But with deep breathing, you take deep, even-paced breaths using the muscle under your rib cage (diaphragm). Take a deep breath of air, pause, exhale, and then pause again before repeating. This type of breathing releases natural painkillers (endorphins) into your body. Deep breathing also reduces the amount of stress chemicals in your brain and relaxes your muscles.

Deep breathing is generally safe, but you may not want to use it if you tend to get dizzy or hyperventilate. To get the full effects of deep breathing, try to do it at least 15 to 20 minutes a day.

DIFFERENT TYPES OF MEDITATION

You can meditate in many ways; here are some of the most common styles.

Analytical meditation. Focus on an object and think about its deeper meaning. You may focus on a passage from scripture, or a concept, such as how precious human life is.

Breath meditation. Similar to deep breathing (see page 104), use your diaphragm (the muscle under your rib cage) to breathe. Focus your attention on each breath you take as you breathe in and breathe out.

Focus on love and gratitude. Focus on a sacred object or being. Weave feelings of love, compassion and gratitude into your thoughts.

Guided meditation. As with guided imagery (see page 104), form mental images of places or situations you find relaxing. Use as many senses as you can, such as scents, sights, sounds and textures.

Mindfulness meditation. Being more aware and accepting of the present moment is another way to meditate. Focus on what you're experiencing in the present moment, but don't react to it or judge it. Simply experience it for what it is.

Transcendental meditation. Repeat a mantra either aloud or silently to yourself. Use whatever mantra is most meaningful to you. Religious mantras may include the Jesus Prayer in the Christian tradition, the holy name of God in Judaism, or the *om* mantra of Hinduism, Buddhism and other Eastern religions. For a secular mantra, you may use the words *one*, *love* or *peace*.

Walking meditation. Want to try a more active style of meditation? Focus on the movements your body makes as you stand and walk. Pay special attention to your legs and feet as you lift each foot. With this type of meditation, make sure to pay extra attention to what's going on around you.

BIOFEEDBACK FOR RELAXATION

Biofeedback is a relaxation technique that helps you teach your body to change its response to chronic pain and stress. Unlike other relaxation exercises, special equipment is needed. Research shows that biofeedback is helpful for managing symptoms of fibromyalgia.

A biofeedback device gathers information from your body, such as heart rate or breathing rate, and shows it to you. As you've already learned, stress can affect your body in many ways, including raising your heart rate or increasing muscle tension. Biofeedback shows you how your body reacts to stress. With this information, you can make changes in how your body responds to stress, which can lower your stress level and, in turn, reduce your pain and fatigue.

Some research shows that biofeedback is no more helpful for fibromyalgia symptoms than other relaxation therapies. However, other studies show that it can lessen pain, fatigue and morning stiffness for at least a short time. Biofeedback may be more helpful when it's combined with other therapies, such as getting more physical activity.

You can learn biofeedback in outpatient clinics, physical therapy clinics, medical centers and hospitals, but devices are available for home use, as well. Some devices are hand-held and portable, while others connect to your computer. Downloadable apps and some smartwatches and wearable fitness trackers let you try biofeedback anytime, anywhere.

Progressive muscle relaxation With progressive muscle relaxation, you tighten and then relax your body parts one at a time. Start either at your head or at your feet and then move in sequence to the other end of your body. This exercise is used to relax tense muscles. It also helps relieve anxiety and stress.

Progressive muscle relaxation can also help you see which areas of your body are holding the most stress and relieve that tension.

"THE FACT THAT MEDITATION IS INVOLVED CAN BE AN ADDED BENEFIT."

Moving meditation

Yoga, tai chi, qi gong and Pilates are all examples of moving meditation. Although more study is needed, researchers have found that these exercises can help people with fibromyalgia sleep better, have less pain, feel less depressed and enjoy life more. Here's a little more on how moving meditation works.

Exercise can help relieve symptoms of fibromyalgia. (You'll learn how this works in Chapter 13). Meditation, on the other hand, can help quiet your mind and relax your muscles. Moving meditation brings these two ideas together. Yoga, for example, can be good for stretching. The fact that meditation is involved can be an added benefit. By combining meditation with slow movements, deep breathing and relaxation, these exercises can improve physical wellness, as well as mental health and well-being.

But research is limited. Not enough large, long-term studies have been done to show that these techniques should always be part of a fibromyalgia plan. It's also important to note that you may need to modify or avoid certain poses, depending on your specific circumstances.

Massage therapy

Massage therapy is one of the oldest healing arts. Massage involves pressing, rubbing and manipulating the skin, muscles, tendons and ligaments. It's been widely used to help treat fibromyalgia.

Some studies show that for people with fibromyalgia, massage can reduce pain, lessen feelings of depression and anxiety, and improve quality of life. In one study, people saw benefits of massage after five weeks of therapy.

Massage therapy has been shown to help treat fibromyalgia by:
- Offering relaxation
- Encouraging circulation in different muscles
- Increasing the flow of nutrients in the body
- Lowering heart rate
- Increasing range of motion in joints
- Relaxing the mind, body and muscles

The downside of massage therapy is that its effects are short-lived. In addition, more research is needed before experts can say for sure how helpful massage therapy can be for fibromyalgia. And for some people, the

4 TYPES OF MOVING MEDITATION

Here are four types of moving meditation. Find more information on moving meditation in Chapter 13.

Yoga. A practice that can help you achieve peacefulness of body and mind, yoga can help you relax and manage stress and anxiety. Yoga helps you focus on the present moment through a series of movements, controlled breathing, and meditation or relaxation.

Tai chi. An ancient Chinese tradition, tai chi pairs deep breathing with a series of movements that you perform in a slow, focused manner. It's low impact, which makes it generally safe for all ages and fitness levels. If you are a woman who is pregnant or have joint problems, fractures or severe osteoporosis, talk to your doctor before you try tai chi. In some cases, you may need to modify or avoid certain postures. An instructor can teach you specific positions and breathing techniques and make sure that you're practicing tai chi safely.

Qi gong. Used as a way to restore and maintain balance, qi gong (CHEE-gung) combines meditation, relaxation, physical movement and breathing exercises.

Pilates. This type of exercise blends low-impact flexibility exercises with strength and endurance movements. It promotes core strength and stability, muscle strength and endurance, and alignment of your posture.

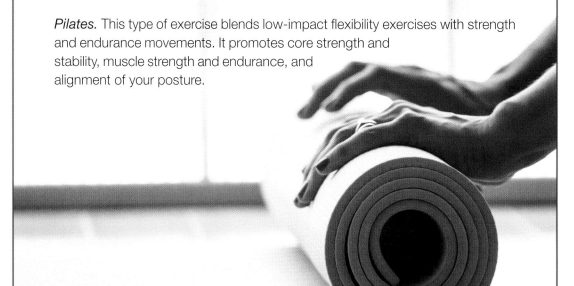

widespread pain of fibromyalgia removes massage as an option completely.

Acupuncture

Within two years of learning they have fibromyalgia, almost 1 in 5 people use acupuncture to help treat symptoms.

Some experts suggest that acupuncture is helpful for fibromyalgia because the location of tender points that are sometimes seen in the condition match up with acupuncture points in the body.

Acupuncture may also help by releasing the body's own feel-good chemicals (endorphins). This helps cause chemical changes that allow for relief of some symptoms. Those who find acupuncture to be helpful say that it helps their joints feel less stiff and helps them move more easily.

Of all the types of integrative medicine used to treat fibromyalgia, acupuncture likely has been studied the most. However, more research is needed because results have been mixed. Some researchers have found that acupuncture helps relieve symptoms of fibromyalgia, while others say it doesn't help at all. The studies that show a benefit from acupuncture suggest that it can help reduce pain and stiffness, as well as reduce fatigue and improve overall well-being.

But to date, acupuncture hasn't been shown to be any more effective than a simulated version of the therapy. And as with massage therapy, pain relief from acupuncture is not long-lasting.

Hydrotherapy

Also called balneotherapy, hydrotherapy involves the use of warm or hot water to relax muscles and ease tension. Studies done on hydrotherapy for fibromyalgia suggest that warm water can ease pain. Warm-water exercise has been shown to add to these benefits by boosting mood and improving sleep. Warm water can increase blood flow to stiff muscles and joints, which can help make it easier to stretch. In turn, regular stretching leads to greater flexibility, helping improve how well you can move. You'll learn more about stretching in Chapter 13.

As with other types of integrative medicine, hydrotherapy hasn't been well-studied in terms of its effects on fibromyalgia. But one larger study found fairly good evidence that hydrotherapy can lessen pain and improve quality of life for people with the condition. This isn't a guarantee that hydrotherapy is helpful, but it may be worth trying along with more-proven therapies and techniques that you're reading about in this book.

Supplements

Dietary supplements are the most popular type of integrative medicine. They make up nearly 1 in 5 integrative therapies used in the U.S. But they're not necessarily the right choice for everyone.

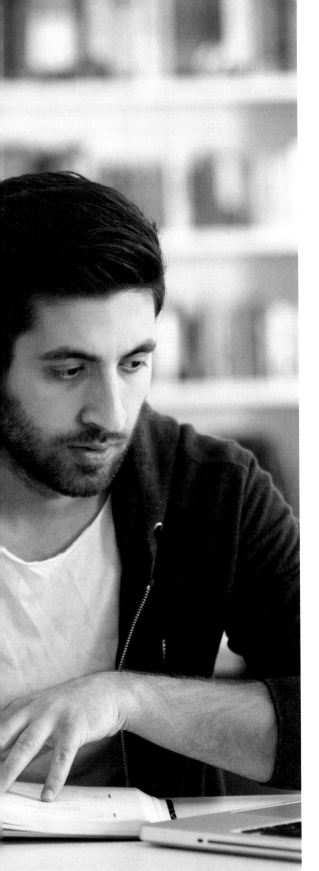

While some natural products have been studied for their effects on fibromyalgia symptoms, not enough research shows that they're helpful.

The only supplement that comes close is vitamin D. Some experts feel that vitamin D supplements can help lessen fibromyalgia pain in people who have low vitamin D levels. But overall, there's little to no proof that any dietary supplements can help treat fibromyalgia.

If you're interested in using any type of integrative medicine, talk to your health care team. Have an open and honest conversation about your wellness and your goals and how you want to achieve them.

Whether you want to try mind-body medicine, massage or another type of integrative therapy, the goal is to find safe options that can help you improve your wellness and quality of life.

LEARNING MORE ABOUT INTEGRATIVE MEDICINE

As with any medical treatment, integrative medicine is not without risk. And for many of these practices, it's hard to say if they will ease symptoms of fibromyalgia because they haven't been studied well enough.

If you'd like to try a specific type of integrative therapy, research its safety and learn about its possible side effects. This is another way your health care team can help.

Your health care team can:

- Help ensure that the integrative therapy you want to try doesn't have unwanted side effects and won't interact with a medication you use
- Put you in touch with someone who performs the therapy you're interested in or who can show you how to do it safely on your own
- Confirm that the integrative therapy you're interested in trying makes sense for you

Finding good research

You can seek out information on a therapy you want to try before you talk to your health care team. But where should you start? Information abounds when it comes to integrative medicine — but it's not always good information.

When looking for good-quality health information, start with government agencies. The National Institutes of Health (*http://www.ncbi.nlm.nih.gov/pubmed/*), for example, offers information from well-respected hospitals and universities. In particular, look for evidence-based studies that have been published in medical journals.

Try to find randomized control trials that have lasted over several months or years. The best ones have included several hundred people or more. Finally, when you do find research that you think might be helpful, see if it applies to you. For example, if you're a woman who's interested in using

meditation to relieve symptoms of fibromyalgia, a study that was done on men may not offer information that will help you.

Finally, when you're sorting through information on integrative medicine — or any kind of medical information in general — keep the three D's in mind:

Dates When was the article created or last updated? If you don't see a date, that doesn't mean the article is recent. Older material may be outdated and not include recent findings.

Documentation Who operates the site? Are qualified health professionals creating and reviewing the information? Are references listed? Is advertising clearly identified? Look for the logo from the Health on the Net (HON) Foundation (*www.healthonnet.org*), which means that the site follows HON's principles for reliability and credibility of information.

Double-check Visit several health websites and compare the information they offer. If you can't find evidence that backs up the claims you see about an integrative medicine product, be skeptical. And before you follow any advice you read on the internet, check with your health care team.

After you've done your homework and you feel like you have the information you need, talk to your health care team about the information you've found. Together, you can decide if the therapy makes sense and is safe for you.

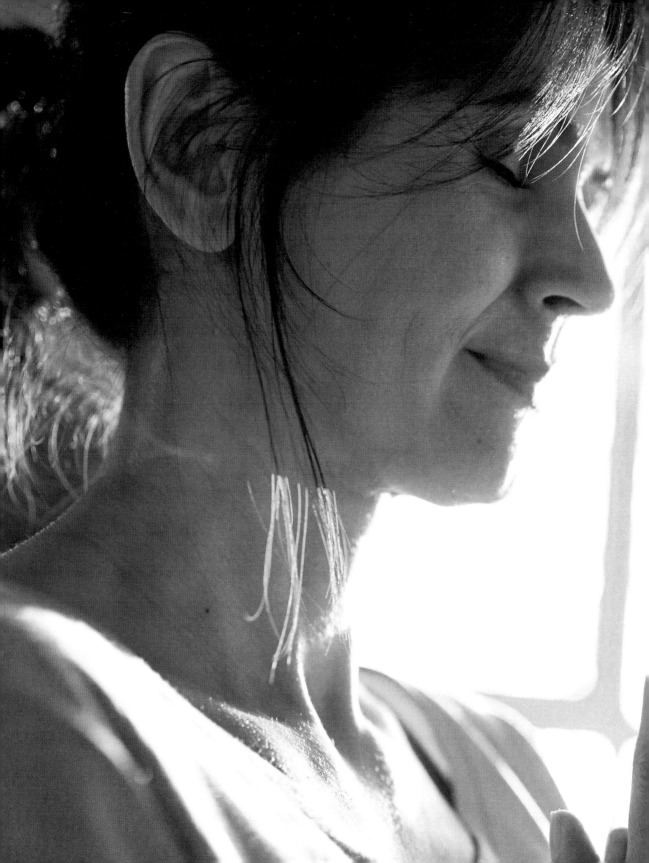

CHAPTER 10

Interdisciplinary pain management programs

Fibromyalgia affects many aspects of your life. So it makes sense that learning to manage the disorder often requires a broad treatment approach.

Your doctor may suggest that you consider taking part in a comprehensive program that focuses on pain management. This type of program is sometimes called an interdisciplinary pain management program, but it's also known by other names, as you'll learn in this chapter.

Interdisciplinary programs bring together several therapies and experts in an integrated and targeted fashion. The focus of this treatment approach is on helping improve daily functioning and quality of life.

In most cases, interdisciplinary pain management programs are intensive outpatient programs, but sometimes they're offered in an inpatient hospital setting. Either way, such programs are usually provided within a major medical center or research hospital.

How long a pain management program lasts can vary, and some are more intense than others. It can be as short as two days or as long as three to four weeks.

In this chapter, you'll learn how interdisciplinary pain management programs work and if one might be helpful for you.

WHAT HAPPENS IN AN INTERDISCIPLINARY PAIN MANAGEMENT PROGRAM

Fibromyalgia affects people in a number of ways. Its effects are complex, which means no one treatment or therapy can address every sign or symptom. That's where interdisciplinary pain management programs come in. They offer a coordinated approach focused on helping people manage all of the symptoms of fibromyalgia.

An interdisciplinary pain management program is different from a pain clinic, a term you may be more familiar with. Pain clinics diagnose, treat, relieve and focus on eliminating pain, if possible. They also focus on reducing the impact that pain has on a person's life. A pain clinic's main focus is to improve overall quality of life by reducing the impact that pain has on someone's life.

Pain clinics often treat pain that affects a specific part of the body. They also treat pain from degenerative arthritis, some types of infection, autoimmune diseases and complications of diseases. Pain clinics offer a range of treatments, including medications, injections and surgery. Health care professionals in pain clinics can also implant devices to help relieve pain. Experts in pain medicine, such as anesthesiologists, are among the main health care professionals found in pain clinics.

Interdisciplinary pain management programs are different from pain clinics. In an interdisciplinary pain management pro-

gram, you're assessed by a team of experts. You continue to work with this team during the program to reach goals that you set for yourself. The goal of these programs is to help you develop a plan to improve your quality of life rather than have someone take your pain away. You learn about different approaches that can help you reach your goals and have a chance to practice the approaches so you can find the ones that work best for you. Interdisciplinary pain management programs are also sometimes called chronic pain rehabilitation programs or multidisciplinary pain programs.

Interdisciplinary pain management programs offer a structured approach based on cognitive behavioral strategies, which you learned about in Chapter 8. Some programs are as short as two days, while others are as long as three or four weeks. You may attend team meetings that include various experts, and group meetings with other participants help ensure that you all learn together — and *from* each other.

Mayo Clinic offers fibromyalgia treatment programs at its campuses in Minnesota and Florida, as well as pain rehabilitation programs at all three of its main campuses. You'll learn more about them on page 118.

The foundation

What happens in an interdisciplinary pain management program varies based on its length. But all of these programs have the same foundation. Cognitive behavioral

IS THIS TYPE OF PROGRAM RIGHT FOR YOU?

Whether or not an interdisciplinary program is right for you is a personal decision.

If you're wondering whether this type of program may help you, ask yourself these questions.

- Is your life focused on pain and symptoms and what you *can't* do, rather than what you *can* do in spite of your symptoms?
- Has your doctor told you that nothing more can be done to relieve your symptoms?
- Are you taking medications to treat your symptoms? Are you concerned about the long-term effects of taking them?
- Is your family's well-being affected by your fibromyalgia?
- Do you feel as if you can't commit to social events with family or friends because of how you might be feeling that day?

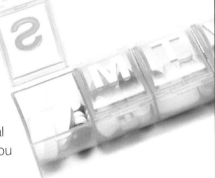

If you answered yes to any one of these questions, an interdisciplinary program may be right for you.

If you think that this kind of program may be too much to take on, consider this. Often, the people who do the best in these programs are those who have been coping with chronic pain for many years. They may have been unable to work for years and likely struggle to handle what many may think of as simple, day-to-day activities of life. They're irritable, anxious and depressed. Their relationships are strained.

Interdisciplinary programs are designed to help people in this position. After taking part in this type of program, even people who have been significantly affected by chronic pain for years can cut their pain almost in half after taking part in this type of program. That reduction in pain is often the start of a cascade of improvements that touch every corner of a person's life.

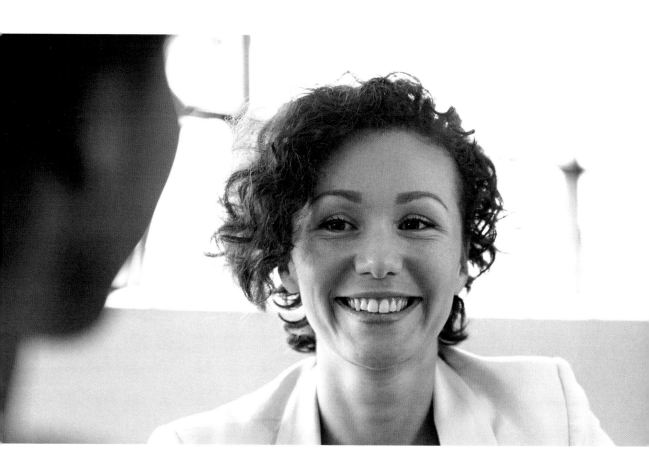

therapy — how you can use your thoughts, beliefs and attitude to cope with your symptoms — provides the framework. Interdisciplinary pain management programs are built around the idea that pain affects every aspect of your life. With that in mind, they offer a broad approach that addresses the whole person.

You'll learn from a team of experts, including doctors, nurses, psychologists, and physical and occupational therapists who all work together to help you. Integrative medicine and nutrition specialists may be involved, as well.

Here's a sampling of what you may experience in an interdisciplinary pain management program, depending on its length.

The program will likely begin with a thorough exam. First, your physical condition will be assessed. Then you'll be asked about the medications you take, your work situation, and your relationships with family and friends. You may need certain medical tests. From there, you'll get help with setting goals for what you'd like to accomplish in the program. The program's team of experts will help you set the goals that are best for you and help you reach them.

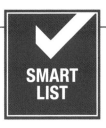

SMART LIST

WHAT TO LOOK FOR

Interested in attending an interdisciplinary pain management program? Look for these qualities before you sign up:

- Beliefs and a mission that align with yours
- A patient- and family-centered approach
- An opportunity to work with experts to set and reach goals
- Treatment plans that are based on your individual needs
- Mutual respect and open communication
- Progress toward reaching goals is monitored
- Feedback about your progress and performance, provided to you, your caregivers, your loved ones and your health care team
- Scheduled, formal follow-up after the program ends

The program may feel time-consuming and rigorous. Some programs may seem like a full-time job for three weeks — eight hours a day, five days a week.

You'll learn how you can use your thoughts, beliefs and attitude to cope with your symptoms. You'll likely be taught these skills in a group setting. Together, you'll all find ways to manage symptoms and challenges.

A family component is often part of the program as well, which may involve a spouse or significant other, family members, and even children. Family members are encouraged to talk about how their loved one's fibromyalgia is affecting them and how they can help make the situation better.

By the time the program ends, you'll have a plan that you can use to live your life fully.

How well do these programs work?

Years of research show how successful interdisciplinary pain programs can be in helping people manage chronic pain and improving their day-to-day lives. Researchers studying these programs have found

TAKING PART IN A MAYO CLINIC PROGRAM

Mayo Clinic provides an evaluation for individuals who are questioning whether they have fibromyalgia. Outpatient interdisciplinary programs for the management of fibromyalgia are available at Mayo Clinic in Rochester, Minnesota, and Jacksonville, Florida.

Getting an accurate diagnosis of fibromyalgia is an important first step. Programs in both locations provide an evaluation to determine whether you have fibromyalgia. If it's confirmed that you do have fibromyalgia, you'll be offered the opportunity to take part in a structured, skills-based program that can help you learn to manage your symptoms and improve your functioning. You're encouraged to bring a spouse, significant other or family member to the class.

If you're interested in taking part in one of Mayo Clinic's fibromyalgia programs, here is what to do:

Rochester: Get a referral from your doctor to be seen in the Division of General Internal Medicine at Mayo Clinic. At your appointment, you will be evaluated for fibromyalgia. If fibromyalgia is suspected, your doctor will then refer you to the fibromyalgia clinic. If your doctor makes or confirms a diagnosis of fibromyalgia, you'll be offered the opportunity to take part in the fibromyalgia program. For more information, contact the Central Appointment Office at the Rochester campus of Mayo Clinic at 507-538-3270.

Jacksonville: A referral from a medical provider is necessary to be evaluated in the fibromyalgia clinic. If the medical staff makes or confirms a diagnosis of fibromyalgia, you will be offered the opportunity to take part in the structured two-day fibromyalgia treatment program. If you would like more information, contact the Central Appointment Office at the Jacksonville campus of Mayo Clinic at 904-953-0853.

After you've been seen by medical staff at Mayo Clinic and evaluated in the fibromyalgia clinic, information will be provided to guide your doctor in helping you to continue to manage your symptoms once you return home.

"PARTICIPANTS INVOLVED IN STUDIES ... ALSO SAY THAT PAIN DOESN'T HAVE AS MUCH OF AN EFFECT ON THEIR LIVES."

that they're more effective than medical treatment or physical therapy alone, and they're more cost-effective than conventional medical care.

In fact, there's more research to support the use of interdisciplinary programs to manage pain than there is for any other type of chronic pain treatment. Some people who've attended pain management programs say they are still feeling less pain and have better functioning and mood more than a decade later because of the techniques they learned.

Such studies are focused on all types of chronic pain, not specifically fibromyalgia. However, fibromyalgia is a common condition that leads people to seek treatment at an interdisciplinary pain management program. At the Mayo Clinic Pain Rehabilitation Center, fibromyalgia is one of the top three chronic pain conditions seen, second only to chronic back pain.

Other research has focused on how well interdisciplinary pain management programs help people manage all symptoms of fibromyalgia. For example, research indicates

that breathing and relaxation exercises, moderation in activity, physical therapy, exercise, and cognitive behavioral therapy are all helpful in managing fibromyalgia symptoms. From this feedback, researchers believe it's beneficial to group these treatment therapies together when teaching people how to manage the condition. Most interdisciplinary programs teach all of these strategies. That's why you're learning about all of them in this book.

Participants involved in studies of interdisciplinary pain management programs indicate that they have less pain, feel less depressed, have better physical fitness and are less tired after completing the programs. They also say that pain doesn't have as much of an effect on their lives. These programs won't cure fibromyalgia, but research indicates that people who take part in such programs show significant improvement in their condition.

The bottom line: Research has found that the most successful way to treat fibromyalgia is with a variety of therapies, performed by a team of experts and done in a coordinated fashion.

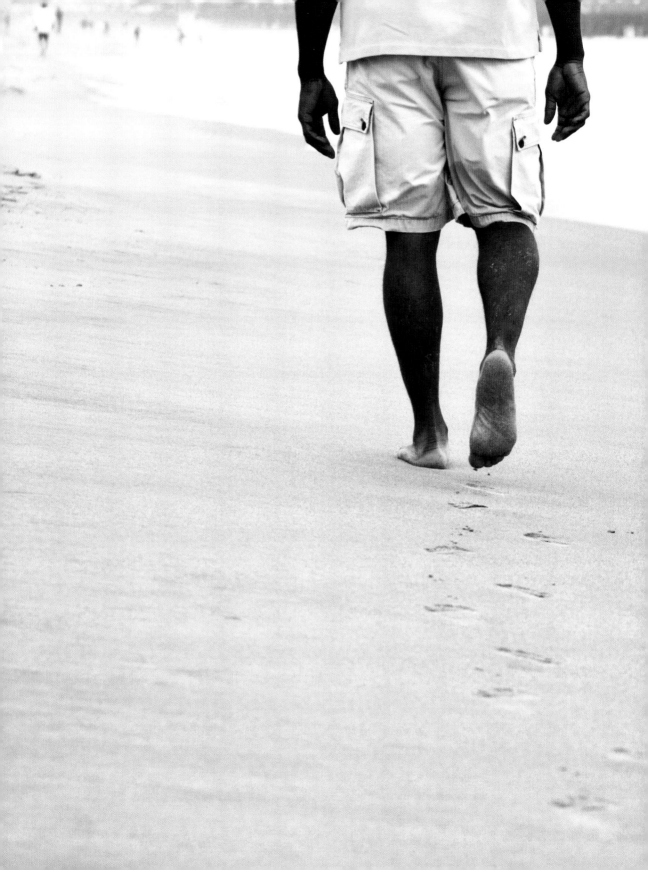

PART 3

Managing symptoms

Medications and integrative therapies are the most common treatments for managing symptoms of fibromyalgia, and they may give you some relief. But as you discovered in the last few chapters, neither approach is considered the gold standard in treatment — the best or most reliable approach for a successful outcome.

Managing your daily routine is the key to living well with fibromyalgia. It involves a focus on your overall well-being, not on your symptoms. As you read through Part 3, you'll learn more about what this means.

In the last chapter, you got a glimpse into interdisciplinary pain management programs. These programs teach everyday skills that you can use to manage your symptoms, allowing you to live a full, enjoyable life with fibromyalgia.

In short, they teach ways to manage the condition by focusing on your overall well-being.

The next several chapters offer an inside look at what's taught in interdisciplinary pain management programs. When the approaches taught in these programs are used together, they have been shown to offer the most effective way to manage fibromyalgia. They're also the basis for a treatment plan that you'll create for yourself later in this book.

Managing fibromyalgia is a process, not one single act. It involves weaving together a series of wellness-related lifestyle changes that build on each other to help you manage symptoms and enjoy life again.

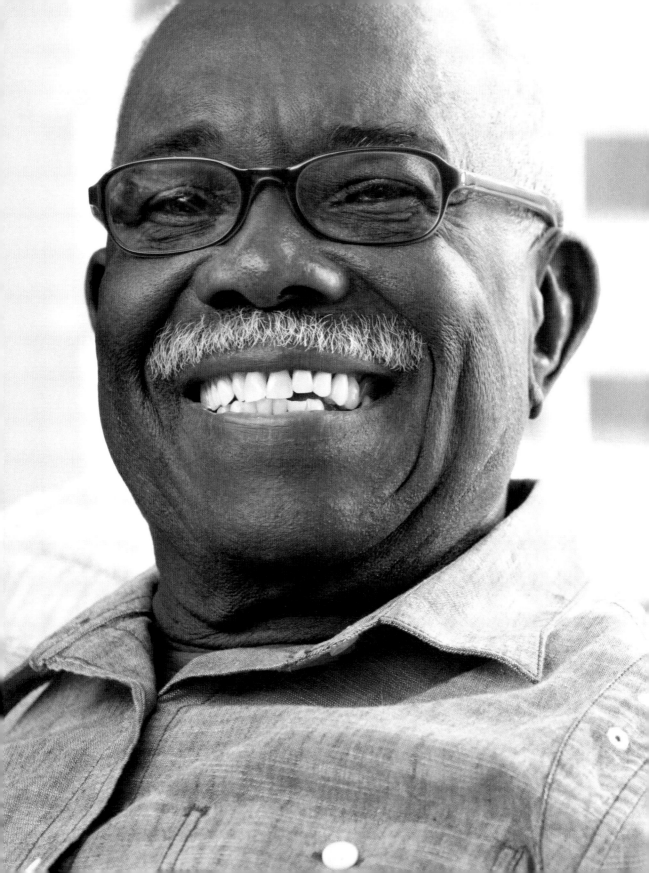

CHAPTER 11

Setting goals

Many things in life take planning. Maybe you've planned for a vacation, mapped out your next career move or devised a way to save up for a down payment on a house.

Just like anything else that requires planning, charting a course for living with fibromyalgia takes active and deliberate thoughts and steps. Planning can help you get where you want to go — in this case, living well with fibromyalgia. From setting goals to the specifics of your everyday life, every detail matters.

Many people with fibromyalgia feel as though they've lost the activities and relationships that make life meaningful. They wish they could get their lives back. What does "getting your life back" mean to you? It may mean going to college or being able to shop at the grocery store on your own. It may mean returning to driving, feeling strong enough to walk up the stairs again or having friends over for dinner. Goal-setting can help you get your life back. Not when a cure is found for fibromyalgia and not when you feel better, but today.

Let's start your plan at its foundation: your goals. What do you miss doing? What have you stopped doing because of your symptoms, and what do you want to return to? As you read through this chapter, think about what you would like to do. On the following pages, you'll learn how you can set goals to make those dreams a reality, starting today.

"YOUR GOALS PROVIDE A ROAD MAP TO HELP YOU MOVE YOUR LIFE FORWARD IN A POSITIVE DIRECTION."

READY, SET, GOALS

Setting goals is crucial to creating an action plan that will help you live an enjoyable, fulfilling life. Your goals provide a road map to help you move your life forward in a positive direction. They help you get organized and direct you toward change. They provide purpose and help you attain accomplishments that build your confidence.

Throughout this book, you're learning that pacing and moderation are important when it comes to what — and how much — you do. The same is true with setting goals. You may want to tackle many different things all at once; it's best to resist this urge.

When you set goals, don't overdo it. Take small steps and celebrate as you build on your successes. At the same time, know that your goals will likely change over time. Set goals for your life as you're currently living it, but keep in mind that as situations in your life change, so will your goals.

As you think about setting goals, you may not be motivated to set even one. That's OK! Your motivation may actually come from accomplishing a goal, even if you're not feeling excited about the process right now.

If you're not feeling ready to set a goal, try setting one that you feel confident you can reach. Get ideas on pages 126 and 240.

Achieving that first goal may kick-start your motivation and encourage you to set new goals for yourself. Along the way, you may get a better feeling for what really motivates you and sparks your desire to be successful.

How to set goals

When you set your goals, the first thing to remember is to be careful. You don't want your goal to be so big that you instantly feel overwhelmed. On the flip side, you don't want your goal to be so general that you won't be able to tell when you've accomplished it.

Researchers have come up with a strategy to help you be successful when setting goals. It's a simple acronym: SMART.

A SMART goal is:

Specific Write each goal plainly. State exactly what you want to achieve, when you want to achieve it and how you will do it. These specific details make for a good goal.

WHAT MOTIVATES YOU?

When you start setting goals for managing fibromyalgia, it can be helpful to take a big-picture view. Ask yourself: What do you want your goals to help you accomplish? Your answer to this question is your motivation — what will give you an ongoing desire to succeed. Motivation is at the heart of your fibromyalgia plan. It's what gets you going and keeps you at it. Understanding what motivates you to manage your symptoms will help you follow through with your plan.

Take a few minutes to think about what you desire in life. Maybe you want to be active with your family, sit through your child's soccer game or finally go on that camping trip you keep promising your family you'll take. Or maybe you want to feel more able to accomplish the tasks of daily living, such as taking care of the laundry. Whatever it is, this motivation can connect your thoughts and feelings to a plan of action and give you a sense of purpose.

Write down all of the reasons you want to gain control of your fibromyalgia. Then rank your top three reasons, with one as your most important. Consider posting this list where you'll see it often, and discuss it with your health care team. As time goes on, if your reasons change, update your list.

Here are some reasons why people with fibromyalgia want to better manage their condition — the motivators behind their efforts to manage their symptoms:

I want to:
- Dance at my daughter's wedding
- Host Thanksgiving in my home again
- Walk on the beach
- Ride my bike again
- Play with my grandchildren
- Not miss work anymore
- Clean my house

A goal that's not specific: I will get in better shape.

A goal that's specific: I will walk 30 minutes a day, five days a week, after work.

By setting a specific goal, you're declaring what you will do, how long you will do it and when you will do it. State exactly what you want to achieve, how you're going to do it and when you want to achieve it.

Measurable Focus on clear, measurable outcomes, and plan to track your progress.

A goal that's not measurable: I want to eat more healthfully.

A goal that's measurable: I want to start having a healthy breakfast at least five days a week.

If you can measure a goal, you can see how successful you are at meeting it.

Attainable A goal that's attainable is one that you have enough time and resources to devote to. For example, your work schedule may prevent you from spending an hour at the gym every day. In this case, a goal to go to the gym for an hour each day isn't attainable. Instead, two weekday and two weekend trips to the gym may be attainable.

Here's another exercise-related example: Running may be physically too difficult for you. In this case, running every day isn't an attainable goal. Instead, choose a form of exercise that's more attainable, such as bike riding or attending a yoga class.

Relevant Choose goals that fit your stage and style of life. Make your goal meaningful and important to *you* — not to a loved one or anyone else you know. As much as you may want to accomplish something because someone else wants you to, the most lasting change comes when you identify deeply personal reasons for doing it. A relevant goal has meaning for you personally. Tailor your goals to your unique preferences, values and motivations.

Time-limited Set a deadline for yourself. Having an endpoint will allow you to pause and reflect on successes and key learnings. And it's OK to change course if you need to. At the same time, make sure you set a realistic deadline. Start with goals you can achieve within a week to a month. If a goal takes too long to reach, you may become discouraged and give up.

In terms of timing, it may be helpful to plan a series of small goals that build on each other instead of one major long-term goal. Setting and achieving short-term goals helps keep you motivated. Find examples of goals that meet these criteria on page 240.

3 steps to goal-setting success

Increase your chances of success by taking these three steps.

1. Take time to get to know the reasons behind your goal. Ask yourself:
   - How does this goal align with my personal values?

HOW CONFIDENT ARE YOU?

Confidence that you can reach your goals sets the stage for success. When you set goals, think about how confident you are that you'll achieve them. On a scale of 1 to 10, rank how confident you feel about accomplishing the goals you want to set for yourself.

1 = Not confident at all
5 = Confident
10 = Very confident

If you find that your confidence is below a 7, adjust your goal to help boost your confidence in reaching it. If your goal feels too hard right away, then it probably is too hard. Break your goal down to something you can achieve. Then, after you reach it, you can set another goal. This helps set you up for success.

- How does this goal get me closer to my vision for my future?
- What excites me about the goal?

2. Once you've identified your goal, break it into smaller daily or weekly tasks.
   - Rate your confidence on a scale of 1 to 10 (see "How confident are you?" on this page). If your confidence level is below 7, break your goal down into smaller tasks.
   - Track your efforts so that you can look back on your progress.

3. Share your goal with someone else.
   - Allow yourself to share your aspirations with someone else. This can strengthen relationships and provide encouragement and accountability.
   - Find a role model, someone who practices the goal you aspire to achieve.

If you haven't had much experience with goal setting or you haven't achieved past goals, don't be afraid to try again. Choose something you're likely to follow through on, and consider getting help from a wellness coach or life coach.

Find more guidance in the goal-setting examples on page 240 and a goal-setting worksheet you can use on page 241.

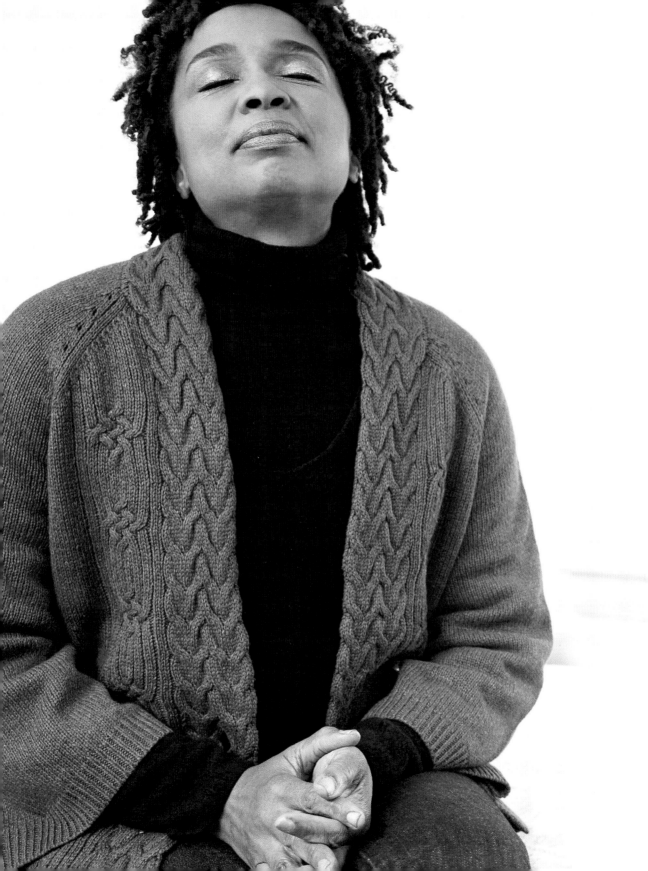

CHAPTER 12

Retraining your brain

In Chapter 4, we discussed central sensitization. This is when the sensor cells in your body that talk to your brain get turned up (amplified), much like the volume on your radio. Or they may go off unexpectedly for no reason. A light touch hurts when it shouldn't. Sounds are louder, lights are brighter. Experts think this disorder causes all of the symptoms of fibromyalgia.

Central sensitization may start after an injury or an illness. Or you may have had the symptoms for many years, and they're gradually worsening. Researchers are continuing to study how and why central sensitization happens.

Two ways to treat central sensitization are with medication and cognitive behavioral therapy. Medication and cognitive behavioral therapy both work by calming your central nervous system. They quiet the messages that your nerves are sending to your brain. This, in turn, helps to relieve the many different symptoms of fibromyalgia.

In this chapter, you'll learn about medications used to treat central sensitization. But most of the discussion in this chapter, and those that follow, will be on how to use cognitive behavioral therapies to treat central sensitization.

CHANGING YOUR THINKING

Your body is continually sending messages to your brain, alerting it to a variety of sensations, including those associated with fibromyalgia — pain, discomfort, numbness and fogginess, among others.

Messages about pain and discomfort are normally helpful. If you jam your finger, for example, pain instantly travels through your nerves to your brain. You react with an "Ouch!" and do something to help the pain, such as applying ice to your finger. After that, you move on.

But sometimes pain messages — or any of the other sensations associated with fibromyalgia — don't turn off. They keep traveling to your brain when they no longer should and become overwhelming.

Research shows that focusing on your pain and other symptoms results in an increase in what you're feeling. In other words, talking about and worrying about your symptoms seem to make them worse.

In this book, you're learning how to change this trend. That's the intent of cognitive behavioral therapy — to shift your focus from your pain and other symptoms.

The next several chapters feature different ways you can quiet the messages of pain and fatigue that are overwhelming your brain. You'll learn how each therapy works and how you can start using each right now. First, let's briefly revisit medications.

Medications

In Chapter 7, you read about medications that are used to treat fibromyalgia. Some medications, such as pregabalin (Lyrica) and gabapentin (Horizant, Neurontin, others), work on your nervous system in a way that quiets the messages of pain and discomfort that your body sends to your brain. They help you feel less pain by affecting the chemicals in your brain that cause you to experience pain in the first place.

Although medication is sometimes used to treat fibromyalgia and its symptoms, Mayo Clinic pain management specialists don't find medication to be very useful for most people when it comes to chronic pain. The risks associated with medication use are often greater than the benefits.

This is where cognitive behavioral therapy comes in. Instead of using medication to quiet the messages your nerves are sending to your brain, cognitive behavioral therapy helps you calm your central nervous system by altering your thoughts and behaviors.

Here are several examples of cognitive behavioral therapies that can help your symptoms. You'll learn more about each of them in the chapters that follow.

Learning about fibromyalgia

If you feel lost in terms of how to cope with fibromyalgia, know that you're not alone. As you read earlier in this book, there's a lot of misunderstanding about fibromyalgia. Having a better understanding of your pain and what's causing it can help change the way you think about it. In turn, this can help improve how well you manage it. Understanding what is — and what isn't — wrong with your body can be reassuring and encouraging.

People with fibromyalgia tend to spend a lot of time focusing on their pain and why it's not going away. This can make you feel anxious, angry and afraid. These feelings only make pain worse. Or you may be plagued by worries of a flare-up. Many things can cause symptoms of fibromyalgia to increase all of a sudden. A virus, the holidays, travel, overdoing it, having houseguests — the list goes on and on.

Knowing that there are tools available to help manage your thoughts and your condition is encouraging and comforting. It provides a sense of hope that can make a difference in your attitude and in the quality of your life.

With the strategies you'll read about in this chapter and in the next several chapters, you'll learn how to cope with triggers. You can reduce your triggers and lessen the effects they have on your pain, fatigue and other symptoms. This is accomplished by learning how to calm your central nervous system.

Adopting the strategies in this chapter and in the remainder of this section may be the best medicine to lessen your symptoms.

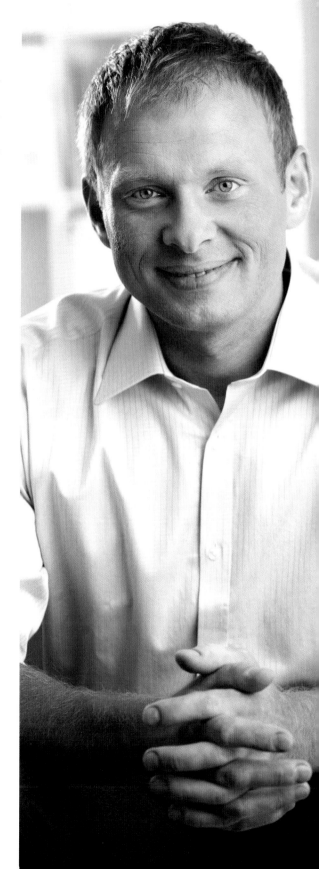

"YOU CAN REDUCE YOUR TRIGGERS AND LESSEN THE EFFECTS THEY HAVE ON YOUR PAIN, FATIGUE AND OTHER SYMPTOMS."

Physical activity

Moving more helps fibromyalgia symptoms. But this may not be your personal experience with physical activity. Most people say that any exertion makes them hurt more and feel more tired. However, research shows that moving more can make you feel better physically, boost your mood and help you sleep better.

Physical activity also changes the pain experience. That's because it activates chemicals in the central nervous system that reverse the trend of central sensitization. This release of chemicals in your nervous system helps you tolerate pain better both during and after exercise.

Research shows that aerobic exercise, such as walking, was the first drug-free therapy to show strong evidence for being able to help people manage fibromyalgia. Walking is often a good aerobic activity for people who have fibromyalgia because it can be done anywhere, at any time.

As you'll learn in the next chapter, the key is to start low and go slow. Increase the amount and intensity of your physical activity a little bit at a time.

Boost your mood

Mood disorders associated with fibromyalgia, such as depression and anxiety, create added stress and make fibromyalgia symptoms worse.

Therapies such as mindfulness meditation and mindfulness-based stress reduction (MBSR) decrease brain activity associated with central sensitization. The practices are designed to focus only on the present moment. Doing so changes how the pathways to and from the brain work. Brain images show mindfulness meditation and MBSR cause changes in brain function, allowing you to cope with your symptoms more effectively. In addition to reducing anxiety, mindfulness meditation affects the pain circuits in your brain, causing you to hurt less.

People with fibromyalgia who practice mind-body therapies say they feel less tired, sleep better, relax more easily, and feel less depressed and anxious.

Mind-body therapies can boost your mood, help you feel more confident about managing your symptoms, and improve your quality of life. Learn more in Chapter 15.

Sleep

Sleep troubles are among the most difficult symptoms of fibromyalgia for people to cope with. Many people with fibromyalgia struggle to sleep well and get enough sleep. Falling asleep and staying asleep can be challenging. Many people with fibromyalgia don't feel rested even after sleeping for 10 or 12 hours. You may feel exhausted when you wake up. In turn, poor sleep can make you hurt more.

Sleep has a powerful effect on your brain and nervous system. Regular, good-quality sleep causes changes in the brain that essentially help treat central sensitization. Sleep helps change the structure and function of your brain and supports your efforts to adopt habits that can help you improve how well you manage your symptoms.

In Chapter 16, you'll learn how you can improve your sleep. Feeling rested can have a profound effect on your energy level and your mood. It can also improve how well you can think and remember.

Connect with others

Connecting with others is shown to be one of the most powerful ways to cope with fibromyalgia. When social support is grouped with the other techniques you're reading about in this chapter, changes happen in the brain that can help you manage your symptoms more effectively. You'll learn more about how you can enhance your relationships in Chapter 18.

Can diet help?

Self-care is an important part of life, but it's especially critical for managing fibromyalgia. Getting enough good sleep, making time to relax and connecting with others are all important parts of self-care. Plus, they've been shown to help reverse the trend of central sensitization. Although following a healthy diet isn't shown to specifically target central sensitization, it's critical in managing fibromyalgia. You'll read about the latest ideas on diet and fibromyalgia in Chapter 16.

GAUGING SUCCESS

The best part about these strategies is that you can measure them. This means that over time, you can look back and see the successes you've had and the progress you've made.

When you reach the end of this book and create your personal plan to manage fibromyalgia, you'll learn how you can gauge your success and measure your accomplishments. In doing this, you can gain control over your symptoms — and your life.

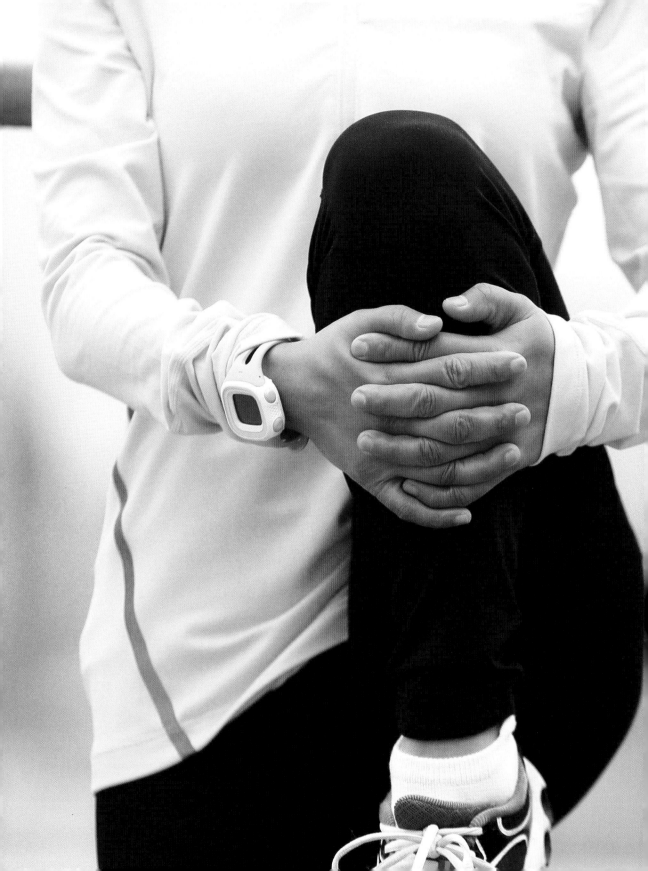

CHAPTER 13

Getting regular physical activity

The pain and fatigue of fibromyalgia can make it hard to want to move at all. But research shows that physical activity is a critical part of feeling better and managing your symptoms. You may wonder how you can possibly exercise when all you want to do is go to bed.

In this chapter, you'll discover how you can move more — even with pain and fatigue. One thing you'll learn is that exercise can actually help you feel better if you do it the right way. Part of "the right way" means not overdoing it — doing so much that your symptoms worsen and you give up on exercise altogether. Slow and steady is the key. Start only with as much activity as you can manage right now and build from there.

You may not be able to do much now, but with time, you'll build your stamina and be able to exercise for longer periods at a time. You'll learn more about how you can make physical activity a regular part of your life in this chapter.

Physical activity is so important to managing your symptoms that there's a spot for it in the daily planner you'll complete at the end of this book. Your goal is to work up to 30 minutes of aerobic exercise a day, but it's up to you how you get there.

Your first step is to find the right mix of activities — forms of exercise you enjoy — to get you started.

"EXERCISE CAN LESSEN YOUR PAIN, EASE DEPRESSION AND REDUCE FATIGUE."

MOVE MORE, FEEL BETTER

One of the most important ways to manage fibromyalgia symptoms is through physical activity.

Even if you can move for only two minutes at a time at first, working up to 30 minutes of physical activity a day is a healthy choice for many reasons. Among them, regular exercise can help you lose weight and keep it off, boost your mood, have more energy, and enjoy better health overall.

But if you have fibromyalgia, the benefits of physical activity don't end there. Exercise can lessen your pain, ease depression and reduce fatigue. In addition, exercise can improve your sleep and improve your focus and concentration. These are just some of the many reasons why exercise is a mainstay of treating fibromyalgia.

While all of this is good to know, you may still have questions. How much exercise is right for you? What time of day is best for exercise? What types of physical activity are most helpful? Researchers studying fibromyalgia continue to look for the best answers to all of these questions. Here's what experts know today.

What the research says

For more than 30 years, researchers have been studying the relationship between fibromyalgia and physical activity. They've examined timing, length of workout and exercise intensity. Today, these studies paint a picture of what seems to work best for managing fibromyalgia:

Low to moderately intense exercise is best. No matter the activity, people with fibromyalgia generally find the most relief from their symptoms when they exercise at a low or moderate intensity. This is especially true for relieving pain, improving sleep and boosting mood. Studies also show that lower intensity activities keep people exercising. Put simply, when exercise gets to be too hard, it becomes easier to quit. This is one more reason to moderate your activities and pace yourself — you'll learn more about moderation and pacing later in this book (see Chapter 14).

It's recommended that all Americans get at least 30 minutes of moderate exercise most days of the week. If you have fibromyalgia, this may sound like too much right now. Keep in mind that this is your goal. Do what you're able to begin with. Then increase

WHY SHOULD I EXERCISE?

If you have fibromyalgia, you likely find any type of exercise to be very challenging. After all, if exerting yourself in any way hurts and you're so tired that all you want to do is go to bed, why would you want to exercise?

Give exercise a second chance. Research showing the effects of exercise on the key symptoms of fibromyalgia is overwhelming.

- Exercise helps prevent fibro fog. Experts think this is because exercise boosts blood flow to the brain, which improves how well your brain operates.
- Physical fitness improves attention, alertness, problem-solving and thinking speed.
- Walking can lower your risk of developing dementia. That's how powerful moving can be!
- Exercise releases endorphins and enkephalins. These are your body's natural painkillers and feel-good hormones. They promote an increased sense of well-being, but even more important, they help lessen pain. They also help you take your mind off worries and cope in a healthy way.
- A moderate amount of exercise can leave you feeling less pain and happier.
- Exercise helps fight fatigue.
- Physical activity helps improve mood by decreasing stress, anxiety and depression.

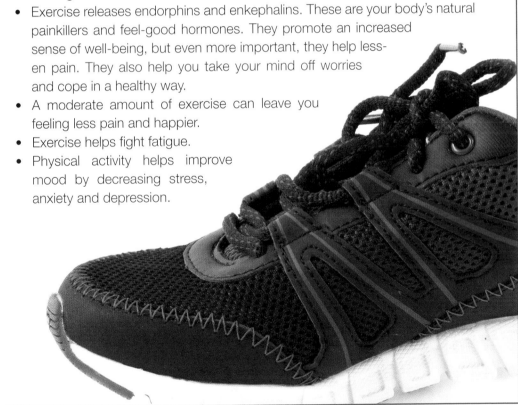

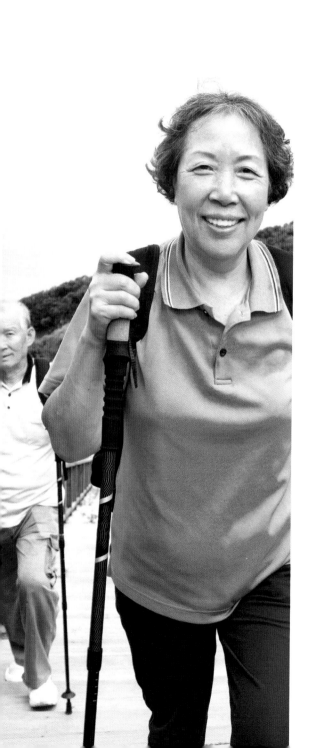

how long you exercise a little at a time. Remember, slow and steady is best.

All types of exercise are helpful. All sorts of different types of physical activity can help relieve symptoms of fibromyalgia. When you're choosing activities that you think will be best for you, think of the ones you enjoy doing the most. All types of exercise — from water exercises to a variety of other aerobic exercises, and from strengthening exercises to stretching — have been found to help reduce pain and improve physical functioning. It's up to you to decide which ones will work best and will be realistic for you to continue over time.

Exercise won't make your pain worse. Contrary to popular belief, slowly increasing your physical activity won't worsen fibromyalgia pain. The key is to pace yourself and gradually work your way up to 30 minutes of exercise each day.

Types of exercises to try

Before you start exercising, and especially if you haven't been very active, talk to your doctor. Together, you can make sure that your exercise plan will work well for you. This is also important if you smoke, have heart disease, high blood pressure or diabetes, or are overweight.

Your doctor may suggest that you work with a physical therapist before starting your exercise program, especially if you're not steady on your feet or you use a cane or

WHAT'S THE DIFFERENCE BETWEEN LOW AND MODERATE INTENSITY?

You can get a good idea of how intense your workout is based on your body's response. Here are some clues to look for:

Low intensity

You can talk or sing easily while exercising. Think of how you feel when you're doing activities of daily life, such as getting up to get a drink of water or going on a short walk. Walking in place in a swimming pool is an example of low-intensity physical activity.

Moderate intensity

- Your breathing quickens, but you're not out of breath.
- You're a little sweaty after about 10 minutes of activity.
- You can carry on a conversation, but you can't sing.

walker. A physical therapist can help ensure you have a good balance of activities in your plan that address safety first and then flexibility and posture, as well as your health and fitness.

From there, use these examples of different activities as you think about what might be best for you. Keep in mind that any activity should be enjoyable — something you'll stick with over time. All of the following examples are low impact and joint-friendly.

Aerobic exercise Any movement that contracts large muscle groups, increases your heart rate and causes your lungs to work harder is considered aerobic exercise.

Examples: Walking, swimming, biking, hiking, skiing, tennis, dancing.

Tip: Walking tends to be a go-to choice for aerobic activity because it requires no special equipment and can be done anywhere.

IS WATER THE WAY TO GO?

While many types of exercise can help you manage fibromyalgia, water-based exercises have been shown to be especially helpful.

Water has been prized for its healing properties for centuries. You read briefly about hydrotherapy earlier in this book; it's a type of integrative medicine that can help treat fibromyalgia symptoms. Warm water appears to be especially beneficial. (Learn more on page 109.)

Although more study needs to be done, what researchers have learned about water-based exercise for managing fibromyalgia is encouraging. Researchers have found that water aerobics are among the most successful types of therapies for fibromyalgia.

Water — warm water, in particular — helps people with fibromyalgia move more easily. The warmth of the water allows joints and muscles to become more flexible and reduces the sensation of pain. Water is also supportive. The buoyancy, flow and resistance of water can help people gradually increase their exercise in a way that land-based exercises can't. That's because with water exercises, your joints don't feel the same impact that they do when running or even walking. Water exercise is also often easier for people who haven't been active for quite some time.

If you have any sort of wound, have severe respiratory problems or are pregnant, talk to your doctor first before getting into a warm-water pool.

STRENGTH TRAINING 101

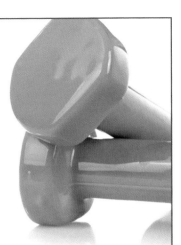

Unlike walking or riding a bike, working with weights requires learning how to do the exercise correctly. A physical therapist or fitness center instructor can help ensure that you use proper technique to avoid injury. These individuals can also help you design a strength training program that targets all your main body areas — legs, arms, chest, shoulders, back and abs.

How much strength training should you do? Mayo Clinic experts recommend starting with half the number of repetitions you think you can do. Doing something is better than nothing, and it's important not to do too much at first. Doing too much can cause pain and exhaust your muscles.

Then, do each exercise slowly, deliberately and smoothly. Count "one, two, up" when lifting the weight and "one, two, down" when lowering. When you can no longer do this, you're done. It only matters that you've worked your muscles, not how many reps you've done or how much weight you've lifted.

Once you have a routine that you can do every day without feeling uncomfortable, increase your number of repetitions by 10 to 20 percent each week. This is something you can safely accomplish and feel good doing — and it will ensure that you're ready to do it again the next day.

Here's an example

Week 1: You think you can lift a 2-pound weight 20 times, so you start by lifting it 10 times, half as many repetitions as you think you can do. Do this every day for a week.

Week 2: This feels too easy, so you increase the number of reps to 12 the next week. This is 20 percent, or two reps more than you were doing.

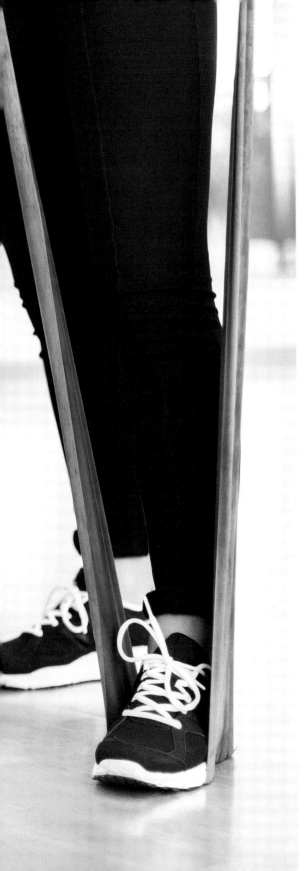

Stretching These exercises increase your range of motion. Stretching makes it less likely that you'll injure yourself. Stretching can also help relieve stiffness, so you can move through your day more easily.

Examples: Any kind of simple stretch; yoga (learn more about yoga in Chapter 9).

Tip: Perform gentle stretches first thing in the morning after you get up. Use the stretches that start on page 242.

Balance exercises These exercises help you maintain your balance as you age and help prevent falls.

Examples: Standing on one foot, walking backward, shifting your weight from one foot to the other; tai chi (learn more about tai chi in Chapter 9).

Tip: Find balance exercises on page 252.

Strength training Any exercise that builds your muscles is classified as strength training. This type of exercise helps make everyday activities — such as carrying laundry or toting groceries — easier.

Examples: Exercises that involve resistance against body weight, such as pushups, or activities that involve the use of hand-held weights, machine weights or exercise bands. Start with very little weight at first, such as 1- or 2-pound weights or even soup cans.

Tip: Just starting out? Try low-intensity aerobic exercise and gentle stretching first.

KEEP YOUR ACTIVITY ON TRACK

Move toward your physical activity goals — literally! — with these tips.

Make it a part of your day. Try to exercise every day. Set a time and mark it in your daily calendar. Prepare to include exercise time when you set your plan later in this book (see page 236).

Take it low and slow. Start with a little activity at a time and gradually increase how long and how hard you exercise.

Add variety. Think of several different types of activities you might like to do. Variety will help keep you from getting bored.

Track it. After you exercise, write down what you did and how long you did it. This record will remind you of the progress you're making and will help you stay motivated to keep going.

Get friends and family involved. Exercising with someone else can keep you motivated and make the experience more enjoyable.

Be patient. You may notice that your muscles and joints are a little sore. This is normal when you first start to exercise. You should feel better in a few days, especially as you gain strength and flexibility.

Moving meditation

Yoga is a strength training exercise, and tai chi is a type of balance exercise. When combined, these two activities offer something more — what's called moving meditation. Other examples include qi gong and Pilates.

Yoga, tai chi, qi gong and Pilates are described as meditation in motion because they connect the mind and body and promote serenity through gentle movements. You learned the basics about each of these types of moving meditation earlier in this book (see Chapter 9).

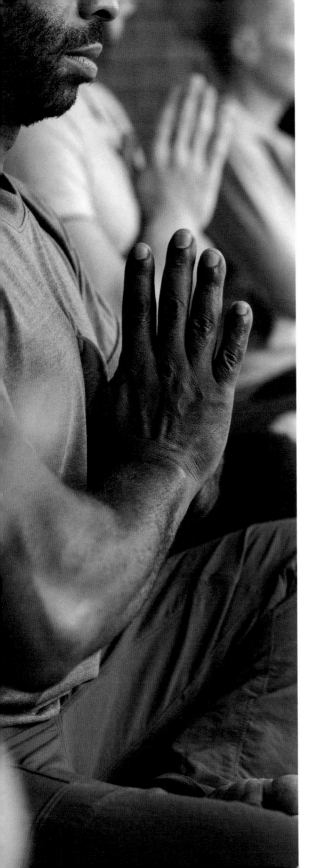

These exercises stretch and strengthen your body, help you relax, and can help improve your balance and how well you move in general. In turn, they can lessen or even prevent pain. The fact that they're low in intensity also makes them easier to do.

Here's more information about each type of moving meditation. Use these insights to incorporate these types of exercises into your daily plan.

Yoga Gentle and adaptable, yoga is often a good choice for people who have a hard time feeling motivated to exercise. Yoga has been shown to reduce stress, improve sleep and even prompt neurological changes that can lead to less pain.

In fact, researchers have found that practicing yoga for only 30 minutes a day, every day, for two weeks can lessen fibromyalgia pain, reduce stress and improve sleep. Another study indicated that the benefits of yoga can still be noticed after six months.

Hatha is a commonly practiced style of yoga that features breathing exercises and meditation. Compared with other types of yoga, this style goes at a slower pace and features easier movements. Hatha yoga has been shown to improve how well people function with fibromyalgia after just eight weeks of practice.

Tai chi Pairing deep breathing with a series of movements performed in a slow, focused manner, tai chi has been shown to help lessen pain, depression and anxiety. It's also been shown to promote sleep. One study found that just 12 weeks of twice-weekly tai chi reduced fibromyalgia pain. Some people have experienced better results from tai chi than from aerobic exercise.

And the benefits of tai chi seem to increase over time: Those who practiced it for several months said they felt better than did people who had done tai chi for only weeks. Learn more about tai chi on page 108.

Qi gong The slow, controlled movements of qi gong have been shown to ease pain and improve sleep, mental function and physical well-being.

How much is enough? Practicing for 30 to 45 minutes a day over a long period of time seems to offer the most benefit. If this is a goal you are interested in, remember to build up gradually. Learn more about qi gong on page 108.

Pilates Featuring nonimpact strength, flexibility and breathing exercises, Pilates has been shown in some small studies to improve symptoms of fibromyalgia. Learn more about Pilates on page 108.

Finding the right balance

You have a goal to aim for: 30 minutes of physical activity each day. How you reach that goal is up to you.

With an idea of what types of activities make for a well-rounded routine, think about what you would enjoy doing most and what makes the most sense for you. From there, talk to your doctor about your plan and get guidance from a physical therapist or fitness instructor if you need it.

Then, remember to pace yourself. That means start low and go slow. Low-impact activities will help you do just what you can do now and then increase the amount and intensity of your physical activity a little bit at a time.

For example, if you can do only two minutes of physical activity on the first day, that's OK. Add two minutes every two weeks until you reach your goal of 30 minutes a day. (Learn more about moderation and pacing in Chapter 14.)

A slow and steady approach to exercise is an effective way to get active, especially if you've been getting little to no activity. In addition to increased physical stamina, you'll feel less tired and depressed, you'll have less pain, and you'll sleep better.

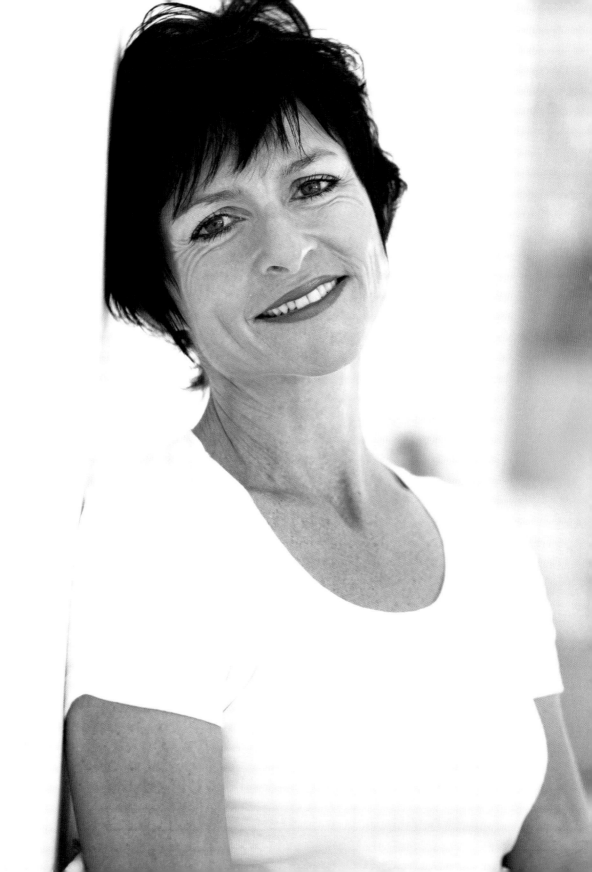

Balance your time and energy

The last chapter mentioned two important concepts in managing fibromyalgia: moderation and pacing. In this chapter, you'll learn more about what these terms mean and, more importantly, why they matter.

You might think of managing your time and energy much like you do money. You have a finite amount of money, bills to pay, goals to reach and things you would like to do with the money you have, right?

The same goes for your time and your energy. You have only so much time in the day, and it's likely you have only a certain amount of energy.

How can you use the time and energy you have to the best of your ability? How can you make sure not to deplete the resources you have? Are there ways that you make sure you don't do too much and feel the negative effects afterward? These are all important questions that this chapter will help you answer.

HOW DO YOU SPEND YOUR TIME?

You've probably had a day when you've felt really good, so you did all of the things that you've been putting off — only to feel horrible the next day. On the flip side, maybe you avoided activity other days and spent hours at home alone, feeling isolated and spending too much time thinking about your symptoms.

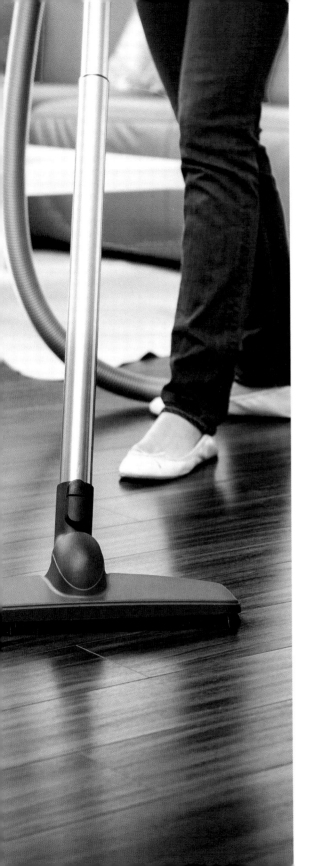

These scenarios paint two different pictures: one of doing too much, and one of doing too little. By balancing your time and energy, you can avoid both of these extremes. Your goal is to balance your day so that you have enough energy for work, family, socializing, exercise, daily living tasks, relaxation and rest. With the right time management skills, this is possible.

Time management means balancing your energy and the activities so that you're using your energy wisely. Time management skills — namely, pacing and moderation — can help you achieve this. By using these tools, you can plan your day in a way that allows you to do what you need to do — as well as what you want to do.

Pacing

You've probably heard the saying that life is a marathon, not a sprint, and that it's important to pace yourself accordingly. Nothing could be truer if you have fibromyalgia. Pacing yourself by alternating activities that require energy with periods of rest can help you do what you need to do — and what you want to do — without using up all of your energy. In turn, you have more gas in the tank, so to speak. You may think of pacing as "energy management." Pacing also helps prevent flare-ups and makes it less likely that you'll do too much one day and pay for it the next.

Are there days when you're afraid you'll do too much so you don't do anything at all? If you said yes, pacing can help. With pacing, you're balancing activity and rest to find a happy medium that leaves you feeling good enough to enjoy your day. Balancing periods of activity with periods of rest helps ensure that you won't feel worse after activity. The goal is to spend the energy you have wisely.

Pacing also means doing just as much on a good day as you do on a bad day. When you pace yourself, you plan to expend the same amount of effort you would on a bad day as you would on a good day. That means not doing more — or often, too much — on a good day. Taking this route, rather than saving up all your energy for the days when you feel great, means that you can gradually and steadily build your physical capacity over time. Plus, adjusting your mix of activities puts you in control of your pain and symptoms — not the other way around.

Once you've landed on the right mix and amount of activities you can do on any given day, no matter what, you can increase your activity level little by little. This may be different from how you approach life right now, especially if you tend to push yourself when you're feeling good and experience the consequences later.

How to pace yourself Before you can set your plan in motion, it's important to know a little bit about which activities require the most energy and which ones don't take as much. You can do this by keeping a daily journal of activities and noting which ones are easier than others. In your journal, you may also include notes of early warning signs that an activity — or an amount of activity — is too much.

Once you have this information, you can create a plan of activities that balances your energy best and builds in periods of rest when you'll need them most. Work toward developing a plan that limits excessive demands and stress, includes periods of rest and relaxation, and alternates between different types of activities.

As you learn to pace yourself, you'll become a bit of a juggler, managing all of the different activities in your life. Every day, you'll decide what mix of activities you want — and need — to accomplish. Anything that requires energy is an activity, whether you're going to the grocery store, talking with a friend or helping your kids with their homework. Pacing those activities throughout the day, or week, and planning rest periods helps you get them all done without draining you of your energy.

Start by setting very modest goals and gearing up slowly. If you're behind on housecleaning, for instance, don't wake up and say, "Today I'll get this house cleaned." If you know you'd like to clean your house, make a specific plan that will alternate activities and won't exceed the amount of energy you have. You may vacuum, for instance, and then switch to a lighter activity, such as dusting. Writing it down can help you stick to your plan and keep you from doing too much — but also accomplish your goals for the day.

AN UNBALANCED DAY

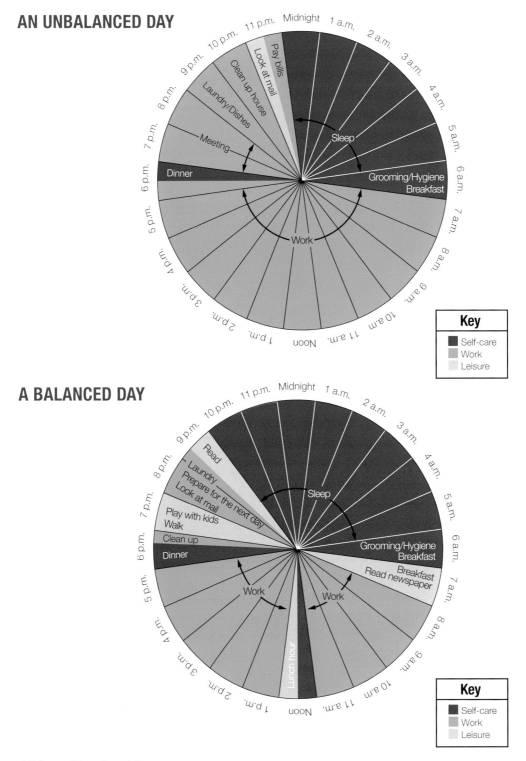

A BALANCED DAY

"SUCCESSFULLY PACING YOURSELF TAKES SOME TRIAL AND ERROR, AS WELL AS TIME. BE PATIENT WITH YOURSELF."

Although you may not be able to schedule every activity in your day, this practice can help you learn to become more aware of the energy you have and how you're using it. It can also teach you how to be flexible and adapt to what's happening in your life. Use the examples to the left as a guide.

You've learned what it means to pace your activities throughout your day. What about those periods of rest you're building into your plan? What should you do with those times in your day?

Resting means something different to everyone. For you, resting may mean reading or sitting quietly or having a cup of coffee. Others may prefer to watch a favorite television program. Your rest time may be a good opportunity to try mindfulness meditation (see page 105), which can help clear your mind and ease your stress. Or you may use controlled breathing exercises (see page 104) to relax and de-stress. Like anything else, resting is a learned skill, and it takes practice.

Successfully pacing yourself takes some trial and error, as well as time. Be patient with

yourself. In time, you'll learn what works best for you and strike a balance in all of the activities that make up your life.

Tips for pacing yourself Ready to put pacing into practice? Here are a couple of strategies to try.

Switch between activities that require a lot of physical effort and those that don't require as much. The idea is to moderate the amount of energy you're using throughout the day. Moderation is a pace that you can maintain every day with no time in bed, and no heroics.

Example: Vacuum and then pay your bills; do some dishes and then fold laundry.

Use your energy when you need it most. Think about the time of day when you have the most energy. No matter what time of day this is, plan to do the activities that take the most effort then.

Example: Have some breakfast, then mow the lawn; after your morning coffee, spend time on the year-end report for work that's due next week.

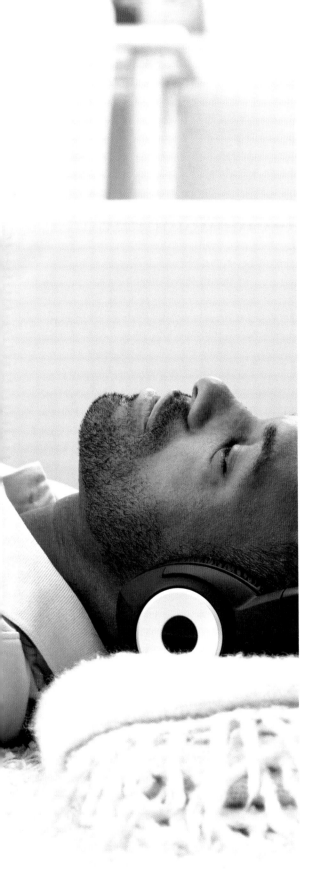

If you have a big project to work on that will take a lot of energy and you have the most energy in the morning, work on it in the morning.

Moderation

Pacing's partner in managing energy is moderation. The two work hand in hand to help you make it through your day without depleting your energy.

Family, work, friends, school, hobbies — with everything going on in your life, you may find it tough to rein yourself in some-times. It's natural to want to give everything your all and not miss anything. But all too often, doing too much can backfire, leaving you feeling awful. Then you may react by doing nothing at all, becoming less physi-cally active and withdrawing socially. You may start giving up all of the things you love to do in life, and that can increase your stress. It's a vicious cycle, and that's where moderation can help.

Moderation helps you take part in and en-joy all areas of your life. A moderate ap-proach ensures that you don't do too much on good days and that you don't shut down on bad days. Research shows that over time, this slow and steady approach helps people manage their symptoms of fibromyalgia ef-fectively.

Take exercise, for example. You've already learned that it's a critical part of managing your symptoms (see Chapter 13), but if you do too much too soon, you may feel more pain and more fatigue.

Instead, be realistic about how much and what type of exercise is right for you. Using moderation when it comes to physical activity can help you sleep better, feel less pain and have a more positive outlook on life — rather than making you feel worse.

Your social life is another area that can benefit from moderation. While it's important not to shut down socially because of your pain and other symptoms, it's just as important not to do too much and feel worse.

Invitations to weddings, baby showers, holiday dinners, work parties and neighborhood potlucks are all part of life. How can you apply moderation to your social life?

Here's the balance that experts in Mayo Clinic's fibromyalgia programs suggest: Accept every social invitation you receive. That may sound like a lot, but here's the second part of this advice: Don't stay any longer than 30 minutes.

Why no longer than 30 minutes? Experts who work with participants in Mayo Clinic's pain rehabilitation programs consider 30 minutes of social activity a reasonable goal to strive for. It helps encourage people to take part in social activities without overdoing it and feeling worse the next day. People who have fibromyalgia often don't have a lot of experience in setting limits, so this guidance helps people use their energy wisely.

Making the most of your time

Now that you understand a little more about how pacing and moderation work and how you can apply them to your everyday life, here are some tips for using these techniques.

Let's start with the basics: a calendar. You may already be using a calendar, whether it's near your phone or on your phone, to keep tabs on events and appointments. A calendar can help you stay on track as well as help prevent you from feeling overwhelmed.

Along with your calendar, a daily planner is a tool you can use to find balance in your life between work, family, socializing, exercise, daily living tasks, relaxation and rest. It goes above and beyond your to-do list and the appointments on your calendar to help you have a better idea of how you want your day to go. It helps you plan ahead, before your day starts, so you can get a sense of when and how you'll use your time and energy. This will help you ensure that you have both of each for your day.

Using a daily planner can help ensure that you have enough time and energy to do what you need to do, as well as what you want to do. Find a sample planner and a blank planner in the Action guide.

Time management is just one part of your daily planner, helping you use your time and energy wisely. Think about which time management techniques listed here can

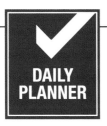

DAILY PLANNER

Planning your day can help you achieve a healthier balance to your daily routine. Include a mix of work, rest, exercise, relaxation and social activities. If you have trouble fitting everything in, ask yourself: *What do I have to do today? What would be the best thing to do today? What do I want to do today?*

Day and date: Thursday, May 10

	I plan to	I did
6 a.m.	Exercise, eat breakfast	Exercised, ate breakfast
7 a.m.	Clean up and leave for work	Got ready and went to work
8 a.m.	Work on letters from yesterday	Letters
9 a.m.	Complete letters	Letters, worked on agenda
10 a.m.	Take a break	Took a 10-minute walk
11 a.m.	Start work on new files	Started new files
Noon	Meet Ann for lunch, relax	Lunch with Ann, meditated
1 p.m.	Continue work on files	New files
2 p.m.	Attend department meeting	Meeting
3 p.m.	Take a break, complete files	Took a coffee break
4 p.m.	Make phone calls, other details	Phone calls, email, memos
5 p.m.	Go home, rest, ride bike	Rested at home, rode bike
6 p.m.	Prepare and eat dinner	Dinner
7 p.m.	Do laundry and iron	Laundry, rested
8 p.m.	Visit with spouse	Visited with Jim, ironing
9 p.m.	Do relaxation exercises, rest	Looked at mail, did yoga
10 p.m.	Read book, go to bed	Read book and went to bed
11 p.m.	Sleep	Slept

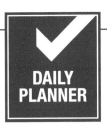

DAILY PLANNER

Make photocopies of this page and use the planner to schedule your day. You can plan a day at a time or make your plans for several days. Each day, write down what you actually did and compare it with your plan. If you find that scheduling your day helps you achieve your goals and live a more balanced life, then continue to do so.

Day and date:

	I plan to	I did
6 a.m.		
7 a.m.		
8 a.m.		
9 a.m.		
10 a.m.		
11 a.m.		
Noon		
1 p.m.		
2 p.m.		
3 p.m.		
4 p.m.		
5 p.m.		
6 p.m.		
7 p.m.		
8 p.m.		
9 p.m.		
10 p.m.		
11 p.m.		

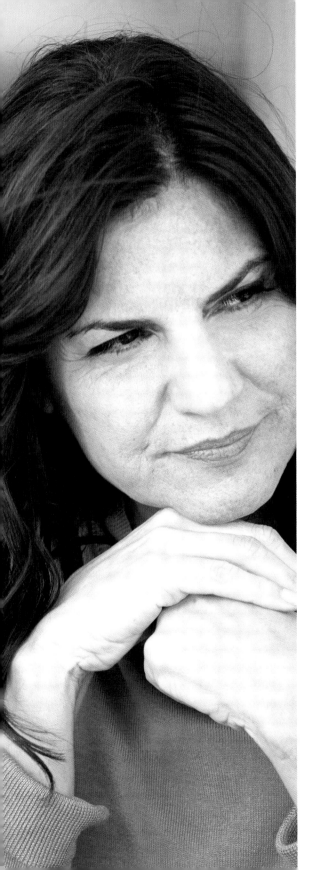

help you achieve balance and add them to your planner on page 236.

List your most important activities and tasks. A daily to-do list can help you prioritize your day. Put the most important tasks and activities at the top of your list.

Make yourself a priority. Take time for yourself every day. Even if it's just for a short time, do something for yourself and don't feel guilty about it. It's OK if not every minute of your day is productive.

Learn to say no. What are your goals for your time? What does your schedule look like? Keep both of these in mind. When other tasks or activities pop up that are at odds with your plans or your goals, say no when you don't have time.

Delegate when you can. When you look at your to-do list, are there things that you can take off your list or ask someone else to do?

Organize. Take a look at your desk and your home. Is everything you need where you can find it? Taking time to organize your surroundings can help you save time and make good use of your energy because you're not wasting so much of it looking for what you need.

Schedule breaks. You may think that breaks will simply interrupt your productivity. But the truth is, they have just the opposite effect because they help you avoid fatigue. Fatigue, in turn, can make it harder to keep moving forward, doing the activities and accomplishing the tasks on your list. When you need a break, take one. A quick walk, a few simple stretches or a vacation day can help.

Reflect. Every month, take a look at how you've spent your time. Did you spend your time the way you thought you would? If not, were your expectations realistic? Did you bank on completing more tasks in a day than was reasonable? Look for time that you can spend more wisely. Taking the bus to work instead of driving, for example, could give you more time to catch up on reading.

By now you've likely noticed a trend. The goal of this book is to help you get your life back — not when you're cured or when your symptoms are gone, but now. There are things you can do right now so that you don't lose another minute of your life.

The tools in this chapter are critical to getting you back to the life that you want to live, to taking care of yourself or your family, and to the activities that you've enjoyed in the past. These tools are part of a plan that will help you successfully return to your life, starting today.

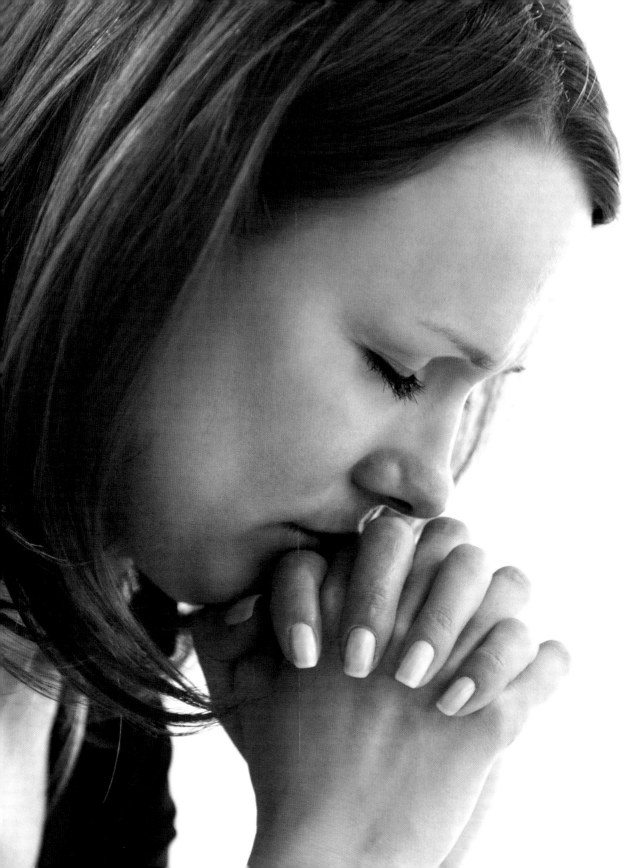

CHAPTER 15

Stress and mood management

Since you were diagnosed with fibromyalgia, have you felt as if your mood has taken a direct hit? If so, you're not alone. Or maybe you've noticed that your mood has slowly gone downhill, along with your energy, as your pain has increased.

Fibromyalgia affects people in many ways, including causing feelings of grief and sadness over the loss of beloved activities or the loss of good health and vitality. Maybe those feelings of grief and sadness are making you feel irritable, depressed and anxious. This isn't uncommon. In fact, nearly 2 out of 3 people who have fibromyalgia feel anxious, stressed or depressed.

If you can relate to these feelings, first, know that you're not alone. Second, know that help is available and that there are things you can do to improve your mood and your outlook on life. You'll learn about what steps you can take in this chapter.

While changing your outlook takes time and effort, the steps you learn here can improve every aspect of your life.

FIBROMYALGIA AND MOOD

Of all the symptoms fibromyalgia can cause, you may wonder why it affects mood. Let's start with the basics.

Stress 101

Stress is a natural reaction to anything that threatens you. Your body is designed to protect itself from danger. If your brain senses a threat, it sets off alarms designed to help.

For example, think of how you would feel if a bear suddenly charged you in the woods. Upon seeing the bear, your internal alarm system would go off. Your brain would tell your body to release a flood of hormones that would cause your heart to start racing and your blood pressure to rise. Your breathing would increase and you'd take in more oxygen. All of this happens because your brain tells your body, "Red alert! You're in danger!" This reaction is known as the fight-or-flight response.

While it's unlikely that you'll run into many bears in the woods, this is an example of danger, which comes in the form of all sorts of stressors. Relationship problems. Difficulties at work. Money worries. Long lines when you're in a hurry. Health concerns. Both major and minor problems contribute to your stress levels.

And stress doesn't have to be negative to affect you. Welcomed events in life, such as getting married, starting a new job and having a baby, all cause stress, too.

Whether you're facing stress that's good or bad, your body responds to it in the same way. Your brain causes your body to gear up to meet a deadline, for example, and then once you've met the deadline and the "danger" has passed, your body and all of its functions return to normal. Your blood pressure and heart rate slow down, and your breathing becomes more relaxed. In most cases, once the stress passes, everything in your body returns to normal.

But what if you never feel as if the stress is gone? This means your brain is telling your body to stay on high alert all the time. This is known as chronic stress. Chronic stress can lead to a host of issues — high blood pressure, headaches and loss of sleep to name a few. Chronic stress can affect your mental and emotional health and even your relationships with others.

How does this scenario relate to fibromyalgia? First, symptoms of the condition can cause stress. Pain can limit how you handle everyday tasks, and this can cause you to feel frustrated, angry, tense and depressed. In other words, just living with fibromyalgia can cause you to feel stressed.

At the same time, stress can make symptoms worse. Feeling anxious or nervous can cause symptoms to flare. Stress can also affect how well you sleep, which can make pain and other symptoms — including mood — worse.

Even good stress can cause you to feel more pain and other symptoms. Let's take work as an example. Getting a promotion might mean more stress, even if it's good stress. That stress may cause more pain, which can make it difficult to do your work. Then, if pain makes you feel as if you can't work,

"THE LONGER AND MORE OFTEN YOU FEEL STRESSED, THE MORE YOUR BODY PAYS THE PRICE."

you may feel frustrated, depressed and stressed — especially if you worry that you might lose your job. All of these feelings can affect how you feel about yourself and how well you work with others. Even if it's good stress at first, it can snowball and make fibromyalgia symptoms worse.

The longer and more often you feel stressed, the more your body pays the price. Your body never gets the rest it needs if it's always on high alert. You've already learned that fibromyalgia, all on its own, affects your sleep. That's why managing stress is important not only for your mood but also for your health and quality of life overall — especially your fibromyalgia symptoms.

What about anxiety?

Anxiety is different from stress. Stress is how your body reacts to stressors. Anxiety describes how your body reacts to stress. While stress is typically a short-term reaction to a specific problem, anxiety can become a long-term struggle.

Anxiety is a common symptom of fibromyalgia. While most people feel anxious once in a while, people with fibromyalgia are more than three times as likely to say that they often feel anxious. According to some estimates, as many as half the people who have fibromyalgia say that they're anxious.

Fibromyalgia produces many physical symptoms. If you've never worried about your body before, you may find that you're more concerned about your health now. You may wonder, *Do I have appendicitis? Am I having a heart attack? What is wrong with the top of my feet?*

Some people may call you a hypochondriac. A hypochondriac is someone who worries about physical symptoms that aren't real. But your symptoms of fibromyalgia are real. That makes being labeled a hypochondriac inaccurate, and it can feel insulting. Health anxiety is a better term to use. When you have so many physical concerns, it's natural to feel anxious about what's happening to your body.

You may also worry about your future. Will your pain increase? Will you be able to do all of the things in life that are enjoyable and important to you? Are you concerned about doing too much, so you don't do anything at all? These are just a few examples of common ways that anxiety can affect someone

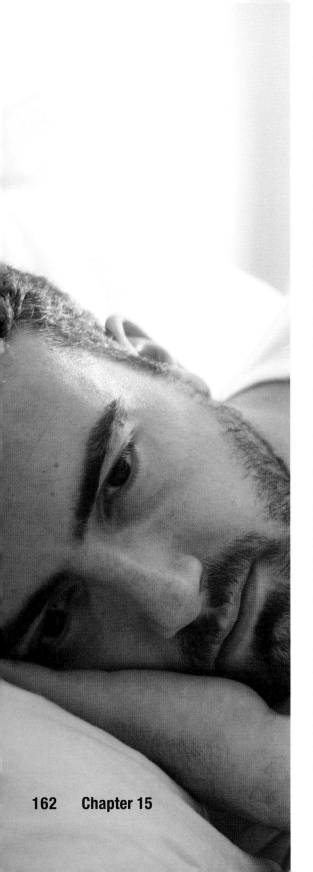

with fibromyalgia. In fact, anxiety can become such a powerful force that it makes every symptom of fibromyalgia worse. You may find yourself in a vicious cycle: Anxiety makes your pain worse, and pain, in turn, makes you feel more anxious.

Ultimately, anxiety can be paralyzing — it can keep you from doing anything at all. That's why it's critical to stop anxiety in its tracks — and you can do it. Researchers have found that by getting a handle on anxiety, you can improve how well you function, feel less distressed, have less pain and, most importantly, do more without pain getting in the way.

Fibromyalgia and depression

Alongside stress and anxiety, depression is common in people who have fibromyalgia. Almost two-thirds of people with fibromyalgia are at risk of developing depression at some point. Although people who have fibromyalgia are more than four times more likely than those who don't have it to be depressed, the fibromyalgia-depression link works the other way, too — depression and other mental health conditions can increase the risk of developing fibromyalgia.

In other words, high levels of pain can lead to depression, while depression can also cause you to feel more pain. In turn, pain can make everything more difficult. Bottom line: Depression and fibromyalgia can be so intertwined that it can be hard to say where one starts and the other begins.

ARE YOU DEPRESSED?

An occasional bout of the blues is something that everyone deals with from time to time. But if you're feeling "down" day after day or most days, you may have depression. Think about whether you experience these signs and symptoms of depression on a daily basis:

- Feelings of sadness, emptiness or hopelessness
- Anxiety or restlessness
- Insomnia or sleeping too much
- Irritability or angry outbursts about even small incidents
- Loss of interest in your usual activities
- Feelings of worthlessness or guilt
- Trouble concentrating or making decisions
- Lack of energy and tiredness
- Increased food cravings and weight gain, or reduced appetite and weight loss
- Overall slowing down, including slower thinking, moving and speaking
- Unexplained headaches, backaches or other physical pains
- Feelings of hopelessness and even suicidal thoughts or suicide attempts

Do you have some, or even many, of these signs and symptoms? If so, reach out to your health care team. Depression is treatable, and treating depression can help you manage symptoms of fibromyalgia more easily.

When you do reach out to your health care team, keep in mind that if you have fibromyalgia, you may have several physical signs and symptoms that can make it hard for your doctor to say for sure if you have depression. Your doctor may focus on other symptoms, outside of how you're feeling physically, to determine if you're depressed. Feelings of hopelessness, worthlessness or guilt are often symptoms of depression that a doctor may look for.

If you feel as if you have no answers or are becoming a burden to the people you love, these may be signs of depression.

Although depression can keep you from doing the things that you want and need to do in life, it doesn't have to be this way.

It's important to note that while depression doesn't directly cause fibromyalgia, fibromyalgia can cause feelings of depression.

Think about it this way: People who have cancer get depressed. People who have any number of chronic illnesses often get depressed. Feeling as if you can't do the things that you want to do can make you feel discouraged and sad. This can cause you to feel depressed. And if you've struggled to find answers that explain your symptoms, this can also feel depressing. Maybe your outlook on life has changed; you may worry now that your life will never get better.

The bottom line is this: If you have fibromyalgia, you may get depressed. People who have fibromyalgia get depressed because they're human — and because coping with this chronic condition can be hard.

Good treatment for depression is available. Depression can be treated and managed successfully. Although you will still have fibromyalgia even after your depression is treated, it's easier to manage one condition than to have two energy-depleting disorders to manage at the same time.

Two of the medications approved by the Food and Drug Administration (FDA) for fibromyalgia are actually antidepressants: duloxetine (Cymbalta) and milnacipran (Savella).

These medications are used to treat the pain and fatigue of fibromyalgia, but they may also boost your mood.

Historically, a number of antidepressant medications have been used to treat the pain and fatigue of fibromyalgia. Amitriptyline is an example. Learn about these medications on the next page and in Chapter 7.

Steps you can take

Stress, anxiety and even depression all have one thing in common: They're conditions that you can do something about.

Here's one place to start: Identify what causes stress in your life and how stress affects you. Through the exercises on pages 166 and 167, you can gain valuable information that can help you handle stress more effectively and lessen its effects on your life.

What causes stress for you? Use the chart on page 166 to help you see what's causing stress and anxiety in your life — and which situations are important, as well as which ones it can be helpful to let go.

How does stress affect you? Next, using the chart on page 167, think about how you respond to stress. You're aware of what happens in your body when you face a stressful situation. The flood of chemicals your brain orders your body to release in response to stress includes cortisol, known as the stress hormone. How much cortisol is in your body can affect how you feel.

HOW ANTIDEPRESSANTS WORK

If you've been diagnosed with depression, the good news is that it's treatable — often, with medication. Antidepressants may do more than just give you relief from your depression; they may also help your pain, fatigue, sleep disturbances and overall health (see page 83).

Many antidepressants are available; your doctor will work with you to find the right one or the right combination of medications. Two of the most common medications approved to treat fibromyalgia and treat depression in people who have fibromyalgia are duloxetine (Cymbalta) and milnacipran (Savella). Amitriptyline and fluoxetine (Prozac, Sarafem, others) are sometimes prescribed. Learn more about these and other medications used to treat fibromyalgia in Chapter 7.

Antidepressants work by affecting the brain chemicals associated with depression. Each class of antidepressants affects these chemicals in a different way.

Talk to your doctor about your options. Once you and your doctor decide on a medication to try, be patient. Take it consistently and at the right dose. It may take up to eight weeks for a medication to work. Keep working with your doctor to find the treatment that works for you. If the first one you try doesn't seem to help, don't give up. Antidepressants take time to start working. You may also find that you experience side effects when you start taking an antidepressant. While side effects with these medications may occur, they generally improve with time.

When you take an antidepressant, you may hope that it will lift your energy and spirits and maybe help with your pain. Aside from duloxetine (Cymbalta) and milnacipran (Savella), antidepressants don't target pain and fatigue specifically. However, they can be effective in treating depression associated with fibromyalgia. Treatment with antidepressants may help improve your quality of life and help you feel more able to manage your fibromyalgia symptoms.

Tell your doctor if you're experiencing any side effects, and don't change how you're taking your medication without your doctor's guidance.

Symptoms of fibromyalgia can cause feelings of stress, and these feelings can be expressed in several different ways. Stress may affect you physically or emotionally, and it may also affect your behaviors. Which of these effects of stress do you see in your own life?

MOOD-BOOSTING TIPS

Now that you have a good idea of what causes stress in your life and how it affects you, you can take steps to make the situation better. Everything you're reading about in this book — diet, exercise, connecting with others, sleep, relaxation, moderation and pacing — all play a role in how you feel emotionally and how well you manage feelings of stress and anxiety.

Here's a closer look at specific techniques that have been shown to improve mood for people with fibromyalgia.

Adjust your outlook

Use positive thinking to reframe stressful situations. Here are several suggestions.
• Think of a stressful situation as a challenge rather than an impossible hurdle.
• Take an honest look at parts of your life that you often think negatively about.

WHAT CAUSES STRESS FOR YOU?

Take a few minutes to think about what causes you to feel stressed. Put the stressors you come up with in one of the categories below. Examples are included to get you started.

	Stressors you can control	Stressors you can't control
Important	• Self-care (rest, exercise, healthy diet) • •	• Other people's attitudes • • •
Not as important	• Tasks you can ask others to do • •	• The weather • • •

Focus on one small area at a time that you can approach in a more positive way.

- Throughout the day, stop and evaluate what you're thinking. If you find that your thoughts are often negative, try to find a way to put a positive spin on them.
- Be gentle and encouraging with yourself. Don't say anything to yourself that you wouldn't say to someone else. If a negative thought enters your mind, evaluate it rationally and respond with affirmations of what is good about you.

- Focus on your strengths and draw on past success.
- Spend time with people who have a positive outlook on life, who don't take themselves too seriously, and who have a good sense of humor.

Laugh

Laughter can help you feel less pain. When you laugh, your brain releases chemicals

HOW DOES STRESS AFFECT YOU?

Think about how you respond to stress. Which of these effects of stress do you see in your own life? Mark the ones you identify with most.

Physical effects of stress	Effects of stress on mood	Effects of stress on your behavior
When I'm stressed …	*When I'm stressed …*	*When I'm stressed …*
☐ My stomach feels upside down	☐ I feel anxious	☐ I overeat
☐ I feel as if I can't catch my breath	☐ I can't focus or get motivated to do anything	☐ I yell, out of anger
☐ My mind races	☐ I feel overwhelmed	☐ I use alcohol or drugs
☐ My sex drive changes	☐ I get irritable or angry	☐ I tend to avoid other people and keep to myself
☐ I can feel myself clenching my fists	☐ I feel sad or depressed	☐ I exercise less often
☐ I have trouble sleeping		

into your body. They're natural painkillers that also boost your well-being.

Give yourself permission to smile or laugh, especially during difficult times. Seek humor in everyday happenings. Read jokes, tell jokes, watch a comedy, or hang out with friends who make you smile.

Manage your time

A day that's out of control can cause stress or make it worse. Work toward prioritizing what you need and want to do in your day. From there, pace yourself to keep life from becoming overwhelming.

Revisit Chapter 14 for time management strategies to try.

Take a break from worry

Refocus your thoughts so that you're thinking less about what's causing you stress.

Getting involved in activities that are meaningful to you, such as volunteer work or hobbies, is one option.

Or turn your attention to something creative, such as gardening, sewing, painting — anything that requires you to focus on what you're doing rather than what's on your mind. Music is another outlet to tap into. Listening to or playing music can provide a helpful distraction, relieve tense muscles and decrease stress hormones.

Take a break, in general

Creating balance in your day by scheduling breaks and carefully scheduling commitments can stop stress before it has a chance to start. Periodic breaks throughout the day can help keep burnout and stress at bay.

This is also where time management can come in handy; completing tasks on time and avoiding last-minute cramming can help you prevent stress from taking hold.

While it's important to anticipate changes and surprises in your schedule — because that's life — you can keep those changes to a minimum through the choices you make from day to day. That includes taking breaks. Experts have found that people who have fibromyalgia and are able to maintain some control over their daily working lives are less depressed, fatigued and anxious. They're also able to sleep better and relax their minds.

When people who have fibromyalgia feel as if they're in control of their schedule, they also feel as if they're more in control of their symptoms. This leads to fewer symptom flare-ups and a more positive outlook and better quality of life.

Lean on healthy habits

Stress and anxiety often cause healthy habits to fall by the wayside. Eating too little or too much, choosing unhealthy foods, drinking alcohol, and smoking are all examples of less healthy responses that people sometimes turn to in times of stress. But these less healthy habits only serve to compound stress. Instead, choose healthy habits to diffuse stress. Here are a few that can help.

Sleep to soothe stress. Sleep gives your brain and body a chance to recharge. How much sleep you get and how well you sleep affect your mood, energy level, focus and overall function. As you've already learned in this book, it's common for people with fibromyalgia to have trouble sleeping. Turn to page 178 for tips that can improve your sleep.

Feed your body and your mind. What you eat affects your mood. For example, researchers have found that people who have fibromyalgia are more optimistic and less depressed when they eat fruits and vegetables every day and eat fish several times a week. On the other hand, eating cured meats and drinking sweetened beverages have been linked to feeling less optimistic and more depressed. Consuming less sugar also may help you think more clearly and affect your mood.

Move your body. You learned in Chapter 13 how fundamental exercise is to treating fibromyalgia. While it's often cited as a great tool for reducing pain and improving sleep, exercise can also improve your mood. Physical activity pumps up feel-good chemicals in your body that enhance well-being. It can also refocus your mind on your body's movements, which can improve your mood and help the day's irritations fade away.

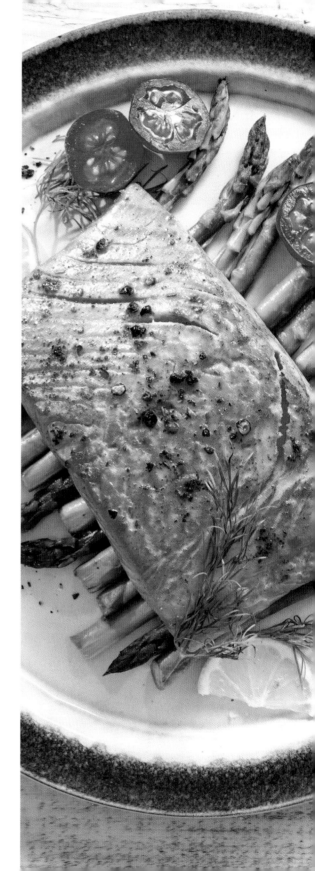

Consider walking, gardening, biking, swimming — anything that gets you moving. Low-impact, mind-body exercises, such as tai chi and qi gong, offer an added bonus by improving mood and relieving depression. Stretching exercises, including yoga, can also help keep negative mood and depression at bay.

Write down your feelings. Putting your feelings into writing can help you release negative feelings so that they don't build up. Just write what comes to mind. Don't plan it, structure it, or worry about grammar or spelling. Think of it as a free flow of ideas. Getting your feelings out is what matters most. Once you're done, keep it for reference or toss it — whatever feels best to you.

Engage your mind-body connection

When your mind and body work together, they can do amazing things. Harnessing this powerful connection can help relieve stress, and the options to do so are many.

Here are a few examples of mind-body exercises that have been shown to help relieve stress and anxiety for people who have fibromyalgia. You learned about some of these exercises in Chapter 9.

Meditation. Meditation can instill a sense of calm, peace and balance that can benefit your emotional well-being and your health in general. Plus, you can practice it anytime and anywhere, and it only requires a quiet,

comfortable space and your focus. Learn more starting on page 104.

Mindfulness-based stress reduction. This practice combines meditation, and breathing, stretching and awareness exercises. It's been shown to be helpful for handling daily stress and reducing anxiety.

Moving meditation. While meditation is often a stationary activity, adding movement can benefit your meditation practice. Research shows that hatha-style yoga, qi gong and tai chi are all types of moving meditation that have been shown to reduce anxiety and symptoms of depression in people who have fibromyalgia. Learn more about moving meditation on page 107.

Connect with others

When you're stressed and irritable, you may want to shut the rest of the world out. Instead, reach out to those you care about.

The people in your life make up your social support network — and social support is the most effective buffer against stress. Social contact relieves stress by offering distraction, providing support, and helping you tolerate life's up and downs.

Talk to a family member or friend about your feelings and concerns. Talking can relieve strain and help you see things in a different light — it may even lead to a healthy plan of action. Learn more about making the most of social support in Chapter 18.

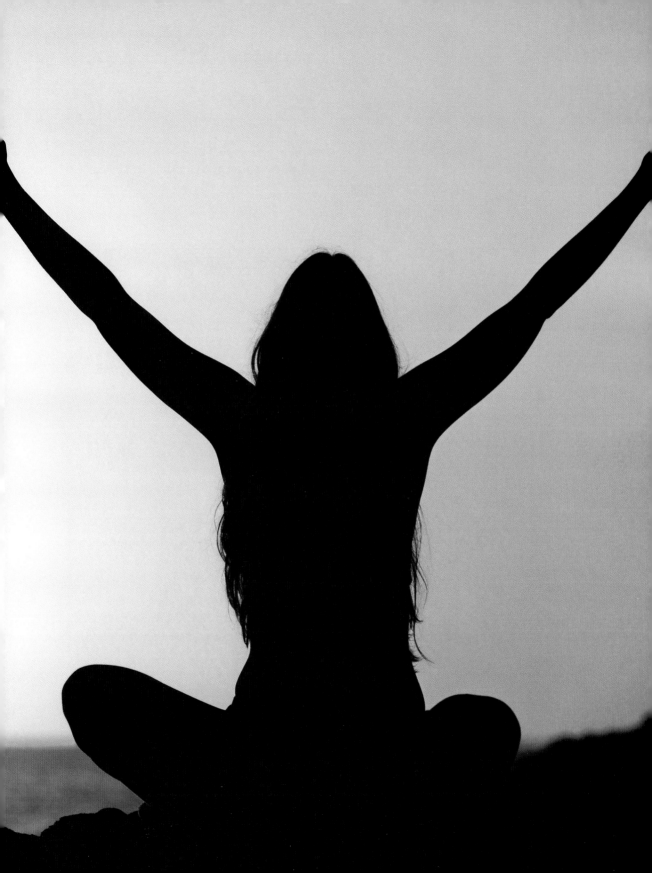

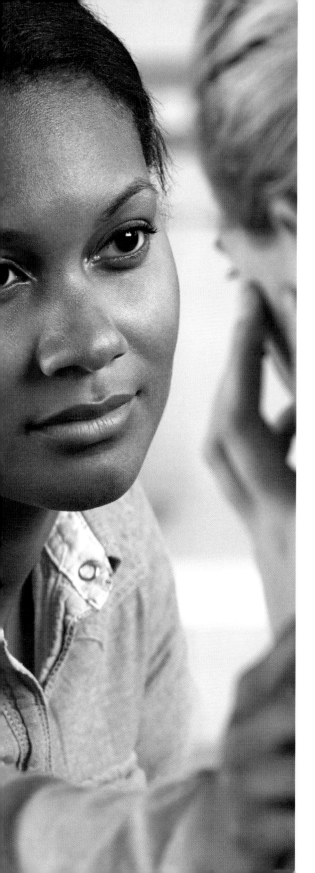

Seek counseling

If you feel overwhelmed or trapped, if you worry excessively, or if you have trouble carrying out daily routines or meeting responsibilities at work or at home, counseling may be helpful.

Talking with a counselor can help you learn ways to deal with stressful situations and feel confident about your abilities. Counseling also provides a source of social support. This is especially helpful if you feel isolated and are struggling with family members or health care professionals who don't seem to understand what you're dealing with.

You learned about cognitive behavioral therapy in Chapter 8. This type of counseling can help you identify stressors and cope with them. With cognitive behavioral therapy, a therapist helps you identify ways in which stress triggers your anxiety.

Once you've learned to recognize negative thoughts that lead to anxiety, a counselor can help you replace those thoughts with more-positive, helpful ideas.

Cognitive behavioral therapy focuses on reinforcing the idea that fibromyalgia isn't known to be progressive or life-threatening. This type of therapy has been shown to be helpful for people with fibromyalgia. Researchers have found that it helps improve mood and reduce anxiety. When it's added to standard medical care, cognitive behavioral therapy is even more helpful in relieving symptoms of depression and anxiety.

Addressing fears, social anxiety and problem-solving challenges are specific ways that cognitive behavioral therapy can help.

Counseling can be an effective way to manage fibromyalgia when it's included in an overall plan for improving mood that includes physical activity, and relaxation and mind-body techniques.

Make yourself a priority

When you think about your to-do list, how do you rate? If you're at the bottom of the list — or worse yet, not on the list at all — there are steps you can take to move yourself up on the list.

First, learn to say no and ask others for help. This can help you manage your to-do list, as well as your stress. Saying yes all the time, to everything and everyone, can deplete your energy and harm your mood.

Second, give yourself permission to relax each day and do things you enjoy. That means saying no without guilt. It doesn't mean changing your life completely, however. Staying active and committed to your responsibilities is better for your overall well-being — but you don't have to do it all. Balance is key.

FOCUS ON WHAT YOU CAN CONTROL

You can't change how the people around you act, or the weather, or if your boss will suddenly decide to move up a project deadline. Instead, focus on what you can control: the steps you can take to live your best life now, without worrying about the things in life that you can't do anything about.

Your diet, your sleep hygiene, your exercise schedule, the way you balance your activities, and your rest and relaxation are all in your hands. Focusing on how to improve each of those areas and letting go of the factors that you can't control can help you feel stronger and happier.

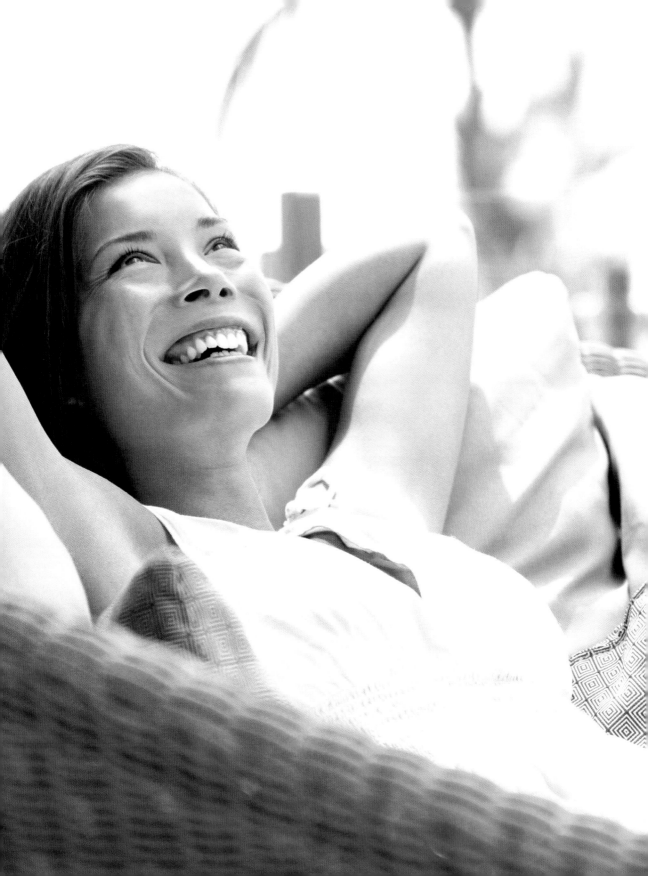

CHAPTER 16

Take care of yourself

Managing your daily routine is key to living well with fibromyalgia. This means focusing on your overall well-being, not only on your symptoms. You've learned that your daily habits can help you manage symptoms of fibromyalgia. From regular physical activity to coping with stress, each small step you take in your daily routine can make a difference in how you feel and how well you manage fibromyalgia.

In this chapter, you'll learn how sleep, relaxation, nutrition and the people in your life can all help you live well with fibromyalgia. With the right lifestyle choices in place, you can boost your quality of life and move fibromyalgia out of your primary focus.

SLEEP WELL, LIVE WELL

If you struggle with sleep, you're not alone. Many people with fibromyalgia have trouble falling asleep, staying asleep and feeling rested when they wake up. People with fibromyalgia often say they never feel rested, no matter how much they sleep.

Unrefreshing sleep can lead to fatigue, brain fog and feeling worse physically. Fibromyalgia disrupts sleep so much that researchers initially thought fibromyalgia was a sleep disorder. Just like you need food to fuel your body, you need sleep to fuel your brain and keep it working at peak performance.

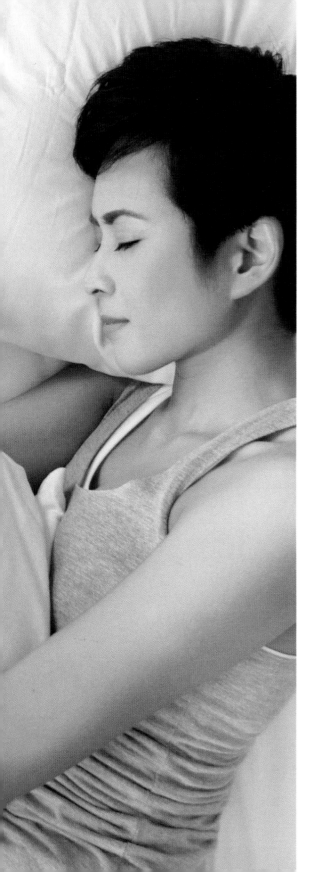

Think back to your life before fibromyalgia. You likely had a sleepless night here and there before you took a big test or had to deliver an important presentation at work. Reflecting on those times, you can probably see how much more alert you are when you get a good night's sleep. Your brain feels sharper, more on task.

Learning a new skill is another example of how powerful a good night's sleep can be. When you're learning something new, your brain is actively changing when you sleep. A good night's sleep helps your brain grab hold of new skills and changes and makes them stick.

These powerful effects of sleep are especially important in living with fibromyalgia.

Retraining your brain is key to managing fibromyalgia (see Chapter 12). As you retrain your brain, you're learning the new skills that you're reading about in this book. Your brain keeps growing, changing and developing new connections, all in an effort to turn these new skills into habits. Healthy sleep is key to making those changes in your brain stick.

Put simply, sleep is the bedrock upon which you can start building a new way of living your best life now with fibromyalgia.

A solid foundation of good sleep makes it easier to retrain your brain so that it's easier and more natural for you to practice the skills and techniques that will help you feel better.

What makes sleep so important?

Does poor sleep make fibromyalgia symptoms worse? Or do fibromyalgia symptoms cause poor sleep? The answer is both.

If you have fibromyalgia, you may feel as though you're in a no-win situation: Chronic pain makes it harder to sleep, and lack of good sleep makes your pain worse.

Even in people who *don't* have fibromyalgia, not getting enough sleep can lead to muscle aches and fatigue, two common symptoms of fibromyalgia. Researchers have found that lack of good sleep can make depression worse, too.

A full night's sleep has been shown to lessen the pain and fatigue of fibromyalgia. But how much sleep is enough? "A full night's sleep" can be tricky to pinpoint, especially if you feel as though you're sleeping long enough but feel tired when you wake up.

Here's the advice from experts: Adults should get between 7 and 9 hours of sleep each night. While advice varies based on age group, this is the guideline for most adults.

To drill down on how much sleep you need if you have fibromyalgia, set a goal of 8½ hours — no more, no less.

One reason the amount of sleep you get is important is because it allows your body to go through all four stages of sleep. Each stage plays a role in how well you sleep.

Sleep is divided into four stages: N1, N2, N3 and REM. Here's what happens in each stage.

N1 This is the light sleep stage. It's the time you spend hovering between being awake and being asleep.

N2 This is the start of sleep. Your breathing and heart rate become regular, and your body temperature drops.

N3 This is your deepest sleep, which is also the most helpful. Your blood pressure drops, and your breathing slows. As the blood supply to your muscles increases, your muscles relax.

Hormones are released in this stage. Among them are growth hormones that help build your muscles. Tissue growth and repair take place, and your energy is restored.

REM This is the dream phase of sleep. REM stands for rapid eye movement because your eyes move quickly back and forth during this stage. Your body becomes very relaxed and still. This stage of sleep energizes your brain and body. You drift into REM about 90 minutes after falling asleep. Then, the entire cycle of sleep repeats itself.

Healthy, restful sleep means going through this cycle four to six times during the night.

Now that you know what happens during these sleep cycles during healthy, restful sleep, you may wonder what makes sleep less restful for people with fibromyalgia.

It often takes individuals with fibromyalgia longer to fall asleep. People with fibromyalgia also tend to wake up more often during the night. In addition, frequent awakening during the first the first three stages of sleep can make you feel more uncomfortable and tired during the day.

If you have fibromyalgia, you also may not experience as much sleep in the deeper sleep stages that contribute to feeling rested. In turn, not getting enough of this restorative sleep helps lead to feeling tired and not being able to focus during the day.

These are two common problems people experience in fibromyalgia. When you feel tired, you may take more naps to try to get more sleep. Some people with fibromyalgia spend 10, 12 and even 16 hours a day napping to try to get the sleep they need. But napping ultimately doesn't help, no matter how much time is spent in bed.

Better-sleep tips

Although getting enough good sleep can be challenging, it's not impossible. In fact, it's very achievable. These sleep strategies can help you get the rest you need.

Stick to a schedule Go to bed at the same time each night and wake up at the same time every morning. Set the same 8½-hour block of time for sleep every night of the week. You'll include this block of time in your daily planner on pages 236-237. If you have the same bedtime and wake time every day, soon your body will be naturally tired at bedtime and be better able to awaken in the morning, even without an alarm clock.

Exercise daily Working toward getting 30 minutes of exercise a day can help you achieve the deep sleep you may not be getting. The key is to not exercise less than three hours before bedtime — unless you're doing gentle stretches or tai chi, which can be relaxing.

Avoid caffeine and nicotine Caffeine is a stimulant that can take as many as eight hours to wear off. Coffee, some teas and chocolate all contain caffeine. Avoiding caffeine after noon is a good rule to follow. Nicotine is another stimulant that can cause poor sleep.

Avoid alcohol before bed Drinking alcohol before bed disrupts sleep. If you do drink alcohol, try to have it earlier in the evening and keep it to a moderate amount.

Say no to naps Naps — especially taken later in the day — can make it more difficult to fall asleep and get the quality sleep you need when you turn in for the night.

Choose your light carefully In the morning, seek exposure to morning sunshine. As bedtime nears, dim the lights in your home and avoid bright light from the TV or your phone, computer or other electronic devices. The bluish light from a TV or electronic devices tends to mimic daytime light, which can make it harder to sleep.

WHAT ABOUT SLEEP MEDICATIONS?

After reading about all of the tips that can help you sleep better, you may wonder if the easier answer is to try medication to help you sleep. After all, many people with fibromyalgia take at least one sleep medication. Whether to take a sleep aid isn't a simple decision, and it's best to talk to your doctor if you're considering taking one.

Medications for sleep are available in over-the-counter and prescription options, as well as herbal remedies. Most over-the-counter sleep aids contain antihistamines, which are used to treat allergies. Antihistamines can make you feel sleepy, so they may sound like a good option. But the longer you use them, the less they work. Plus, they can cause dry mouth, dizziness and daytime sleepiness.

If you're interested in trying a prescription medication to help you sleep better, talk to your doctor. These medications, too, aren't recommended for long-term use. They can cause daytime drowsiness and increase your risk of falling. These medications can also become habit-forming.

Other types of prescription medications have been said to help improve sleep for people who have fibromyalgia. They include amitriptyline, which is an antidepressant, and pregabalin (Lyrica). Again, it's important to weigh the pros and cons of any medication with your doctor.

Learn more about these medications in Chapter 7.

It's also important to note that if you take a sleep medication and then stop taking it, you'll probably notice that your sleep is temporarily disrupted. This is called rebound effect. It will resolve with time, but it can be concerning when it does happen. Work with your doctor to slowly decrease your use of the medication over time to lessen this effect.

Melatonin and valerian are dietary supplements that are sometimes used as sleep aids. Melatonin is considered safe to use for a few weeks, but it hasn't been studied thoroughly for long-term use. Melatonin therapy seems to be the most helpful for people who have an issue with their circadian rhythm, which regulates when they wake and when they sleep.

Also, it's unclear just how well melatonin can treat insomnia alone. Valerian also hasn't been well-studied for treating insomnia. Using it in high doses or for too long may be linked to liver damage.

Why does this matter? It all comes down to the melatonin in your body.

Melatonin is a hormone released by the brain in the evening. It helps start the process of sleep. The release of melatonin into your body is tied to your body's normal circadian rhythm. In short, melatonin decreases when you're exposed to daylight, and it increases when it gets dark at night.

The bluish light from a TV or from electronic devices mimics daylight. This causes less melatonin to be released into your body and makes it harder to sleep.

Relax Do something relaxing before bed. Reading a book, listening to music or taking a warm bath are all options to try.

Double-check your medications Some over-the-counter and prescription medications can cause sleep problems. Talk to your doctor to find out if you're taking medications that might interfere with your sleep. Or find out if you can take your medication earlier in the day if it's making it harder for you to sleep.

People who are motivated to improve their sleep have been shown to get more sleep than people who aren't as committed to making it happen. Even people who have chronic pain get better sleep if they embrace the idea that a regular bedtime is important.

Your first step toward getting better sleep may simply be to *commit* to changing your sleep habits.

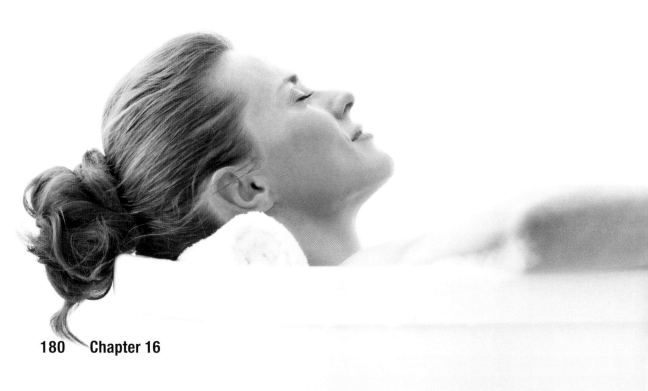

Once you've committed to following a sleep schedule and sticking to some sensible sleep guidelines — often called sleep hygiene — take a closer look at your bedroom. Is your mattress comfortable? Do you have the right pillow? Is your room quiet and dark? Do you have your thermostat set to the right temperature?

With chronic pain, you may be more sensitive to noise, light or temperature. That's why creating a cool, dark, quiet space for sleep matters. The more you can do to set yourself up for a good night's sleep, the more successful you'll be.

By practicing these tips, you'll be on your way to better sleep — and feeling better during the day, too.

Options beyond sleep hygiene

If you still find that you're not sleeping well after trying the tips you've read about so far in this chapter, these strategies may be worth a try.

Try cognitive behavioral therapy As you learned earlier, cognitive behavioral therapy is based on the idea that you can use your thoughts, beliefs and attitude to cope with your symptoms. It's one more tool that can improve how well you sleep.

Cognitive behavioral therapy targets the thoughts and beliefs that may be keeping you from sleeping well. On the next page, you'll find examples of thoughts that may be keeping you from getting good sleep.

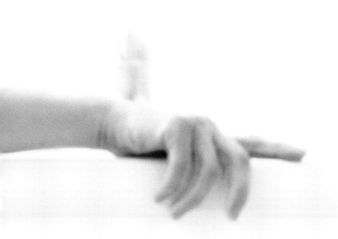

I feel so tired. I think I'll spend a little more time in bed today.

If I just try harder, I'll sleep better.

I'm so tired today. I'll just drink another cup of coffee to get me going this morning.

If these sound familiar to you, take heart. Recognizing the thoughts and ideas that may be hindering good sleep is the first step toward changing your thoughts and sleeping better. By recognizing the thoughts, beliefs and attitudes that are keeping you from sleeping well, you can work toward changing them.

Researchers have found that cognitive behavioral therapy helps improve sleep. It works so well, in fact, that it's generally recommended as the first line of treatment for the sleep disruption that so many people with fibromyalgia experience. It's been shown to work as well — and even better — than sleep medications.

In one study, for example, researchers found that women with fibromyalgia who used cognitive behavioral therapy not only slept better but also had less pain, felt less depressed, were less anxious and could function better during the day.

Cognitive behavioral therapy offers other benefits, too — namely, it doesn't have side effects like sleep medications do. If you're interested in trying cognitive behavioral therapy for your insomnia, talk to your health care team.

Relax Doing something relaxing before bedtime is a good tip for better sleep. The more you can reduce stress, the better you'll feel — and in turn, the better you'll sleep. This is where planned relaxation — 20 minutes, twice a day — enters the picture.

Planned relaxation is such an important part of your daily plan to manage your symptoms that there's a place for it in the daily planner you'll complete at the end of this book.

When you take time to relax, you're actively reducing the stress that's contributing to your pain, fatigue and mood disturbances. Learning to relax helps release the tension in your muscles and prevent muscle spasms. You'll have more energy for daily tasks, be able to focus better and feel more able to tackle challenges that come your way.

All of this is possible just by taking time to relax. And all of this, in turn, will help you sleep better at night.

Structured relaxation helps relieve stress by invoking the relaxation response. This is the opposite of the fight-or-flight response you experience when you face stress. Instead of gearing up to cope with stress, relaxation helps your body and mind slow down.

Relaxation exercises help lower your heart rate, blood pressure and breathing, send more blood to your brain, and relieve tension in your muscles. In essence, relaxation exercises help you send a message of calm to your brain.

You can use a variety of relaxation exercises to fill your time — again, 20 minutes, twice a day. If you need ideas for relaxation exercises to try, turn to page 254. Once you decide which ones you want to try, add them to your daily planner on pages 236-237.

If you try one but it doesn't work for you, keep trying until you find the exercises that help you most. Also, remember that learning to relax takes practice, so be patient with yourself. In time, you'll learn this new skill and reap its benefits. Simply taking slow, deep breaths may be a good place to start.

With any relaxation exercise you use, a few tips can help you set the stage for success. Here are a few starting points: Dim the lights, choose a quiet space and find a comfortable chair. Loosen any tightfitting clothing and remove any distracting jewelry.

HEALING POWER OF HEALTHY EATING

A diet that's rich in nutrients, vitamins and minerals can improve how well you feel. While no specific diet has been shown to be effective for relieving symptoms of fibromyalgia, healthy-eating habits are one way to nurture your wellness.

A healthy diet can be a challenge for people who have fibromyalgia. Half of people with fibromyalgia, for example, also have irritable bowel syndrome (IBS). IBS is a disorder that causes chronic belly pain and a change in bowel habits. If you have IBS, you'll find

tips to help you on page 188. Many other people with fibromyalgia have other stomach issues and are sensitive to certain foods.

No one diet has been shown to work well for everyone with fibromyalgia. However, these healthy-eating suggestions may be worth considering:

• Eat a variety of foods.
• Base your diet on fruits, vegetables and whole grains.
• Limit saturated fat, cholesterol, sugar and salt.
• Keep your portions moderate.
• Drink plenty of water.
• Limit caffeinated and alcoholic beverages.

Researchers have uncovered other tips that may be helpful as well. For example, avoiding sugar spikes can help keep fatigue at bay. Some research has shown that vegetarian diets appear to be helpful in reducing fibromyalgia pain. Your diet can affect your mood, too.

Research has shown, for example, that women with fibromyalgia who ate fruits and vegetables every day and fish several times a week felt more hopeful and less depressed. On the flip side, women in the same study felt less hopeful and more depressed when they consumed cured meats and sugary beverages on a regular basis.

Some people with fibromyalgia find that their symptoms worsen after they eat certain foods. Dairy products, eggs, gluten, processed foods and red meat are all examples of common problem foods.

REACH AND MAINTAIN A HEALTHY WEIGHT

Although weight gain isn't seen as a direct cause of fibromyalgia, researchers continue to look into the role obesity may play in the condition. Some research shows that being overweight may increase the risk of widespread pain that's common in fibromyalgia. Some researchers have gone so far as to say that obesity may actually increase the risk of fibromyalgia, especially in women who don't get much physical activity. But more research is needed to understand the link between obesity and fibromyalgia.

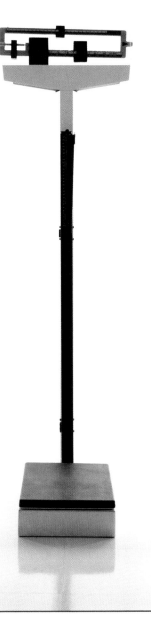

Reaching and maintaining a healthy weight can be especially helpful with fibromyalgia. Researchers have found that people who are overweight and have fibromyalgia are more likely to be affected by pain and fatigue. On the flip side, losing weight can improve nearly every symptom of fibromyalgia. A healthy weight can:

- Improve your flexibility
- Decrease stress on your muscles and joints
- Make it easier to manage pain and other symptoms
- Give you more energy
- Reduce pain and sensitivity
- Improve feelings of depression

If you think you're sensitive to certain foods, it may be helpful to eliminate the ones you believe to be culprits for two to four weeks and see if you feel better. Then, gradually add those foods back and see how you feel.

A food journal can help you track what you've eaten and any reaction you've had. The key with any healthy-eating choice is to be able to incorporate it into your lifestyle long term.

Tips for improving your diet

Ready to put what you've learned about good nutrition into practice? Take these steps to get started.

Keep a food journal Keeping a food journal can help you identify eating patterns that you'd like to change.

For example, maybe you realize that the choices you make aren't as healthy when you're stressed. And as you've already learned, keeping a journal can help you identify foods you may be sensitive to.

Start by writing down what you eat and how you feel afterward. You may find that some foods make pain worse or make you feel more tired. On the other hand, you may find that other foods and food combinations make you feel better and give you a boost of energy.

Drink plenty of water Even mild dehydration can affect your memory and in-crease anxiety and fatigue. Drinking plenty of water offers many benefits; among them, it helps ease headaches and backaches. Keep a water bottle handy to help you remember to drink water throughout the day.

Think protein for breakfast Breakfast is a healthy habit to adopt for a number of reasons. Specifically, starting your day with protein and whole grains — say, oatmeal and a soft-boiled egg — can help keep your blood glucose from spiking, which helps control fatigue.

Eat on a schedule Eating meals at regular times throughout the day can help regulate your internal clock. This can help you sleep better and, in turn, prevent fatigue.

Use a small plate This will help you control how much you eat, which will help you manage your weight.

Keep healthy snacks visible on the counter or in your refrigerator.

"Out of sight, out of mind" is true when it comes to healthy eating. If you can't easily find healthy foods, you may be less likely to choose them. Research shows that simply changing out a candy bowl for a fruit bowl, for instance, helps curb sugary snacking.

Stop eating alone at your desk If you work in an office, you may be one of the millions of Americans who eats meals at a desk.

FOODS TO EAT AND AVOID

Food won't magically cure fibromyalgia symptoms, but what you eat can make a difference in how you feel.

Some foods are packed with extra nutritional value. These foods may be helpful for people with fibromyalgia.

- **Salmon.** Salmon and other cold-water fish, such as lake trout, herring, sardines and tuna, contain the most omega-3 fatty acids.
- **Black beans.** Magnesium helps maintain nerve and muscle function, and black beans are high in magnesium. Other types of beans, as well as nuts, seeds, whole grains, milk and yogurt, also are good sources of magnesium.

- **Dark, leafy greens.** Rich in calcium and antioxidants, dark, leafy greens such as Swiss chard, kale, mustard greens, collards and spinach have been shown to help improve fibromyalgia symptoms.
- **Nuts and seeds.** Like cold-water fish, walnuts, almonds and flaxseed also contain healthy omega-3 fatty acids.
- **Colorful fruits and veggies.** Fruits and vegetables — the more colorful, the better — can boost the antioxidants in your body. Antioxidants support good health in general and have been tied to helping prevent or at least slow down the progression of several conditions, including fibromyalgia. They've also been shown to reduce fibromyalgia symptoms.

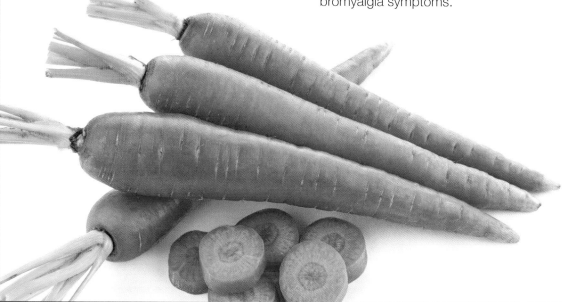

What about foods to avoid? Some research shows that limiting these in your diet may be helpful.

- **High-fructose corn syrup.** Some researchers believe that high-fructose corn syrup may trigger fibromyalgia symptoms. Many processed and snack foods contain high-fructose corn syrup, as do sodas and other sweetened beverages.

- **Caffeine.** It may be good to limit caffeine in any form. You've learned about the sleep problems that drinking coffee can cause. Caffeine also has been shown to cause your body to lose calcium more quickly than you can replace it. This can place stress on your adrenal glands. These glands release adrenaline, which can cause fibromyalgia symptoms to flare up.

- **MSG.** A flavor enhancer commonly added to many fast foods and packaged foods, monosodium glutamate has been shown to cause insomnia.

- **Salt.** One of the many health hazards of too much salt is that it can cause your muscles to feel tight.

- **Sugar.** Some people who have fibromyalgia say that they feel better when they limit the sugar in their diet. Too much sugar can cause fatigue.

- **Dairy products.** Some studies have found that avoiding dairy products improves fibromyalgia symptoms.

- **Unhealthy fats.** Not all fats are created equal. Trans fats, used in cooking deep-fried foods, for example, can make fibromyalgia symptoms worse. A high-fat diet, in general, may lead to more pain.

- **Aspartame.** Found in some artificial sweeteners, aspartame has caused muscle pain in rare cases.

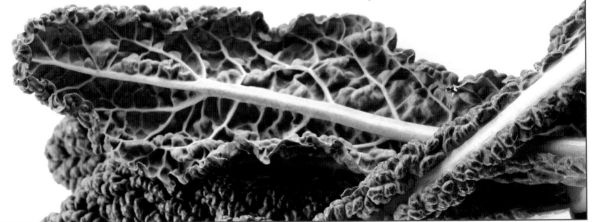

WHAT IF YOU HAVE IRRITABLE BOWEL SYNDROME?

Irritable bowel syndrome (IBS) is common among people who have fibromyalgia. Between one-third to one-half of people who have fibromyalgia have IBS, too.

If you have IBS, you know that its signs and symptoms — belly pain or cramping, bloating, gas, diarrhea and constipation — can make it difficult to figure out which foods will make you feel better and which ones will make you feel worse.

But what if you didn't have to focus entirely on food when coping with IBS? Researchers have learned that there's another way to manage IBS symptoms. Studies show that IBS has the same cause as fibromyalgia does: central sensitization (learn more in Chapters 4 and 5). That means that the strategies you're learning that calm the central nervous system and help manage your fibromyalgia can help with IBS, too.

Conventional treatment is certainly one way to treat IBS. Fiber supplements, a variety of medications and lifestyle changes, and diet can help treat IBS. Several different types of integrative medicine, including probiotics, peppermint and fennel fruits, may help, too.

But because IBS is caused by central sensitization, strategies that help calm the central nervous system can also be helpful (see Chapter 12). Cognitive behavioral therapy, regular exercise, yoga, meditation, progressive relaxation exercises and deep-breathing exercises are all examples.

Almost two-thirds of working adults do. Instead, take a true lunch break. Use this time to connect with your co-workers. This practice can improve your attitude *and* your symptoms. It may also help keep you from overeating.

CONNECTING WITH OTHERS

Later in this book, you'll read about how your family, other loved ones and friends play an important role in helping you manage fibromyalgia. You'll also learn ways that

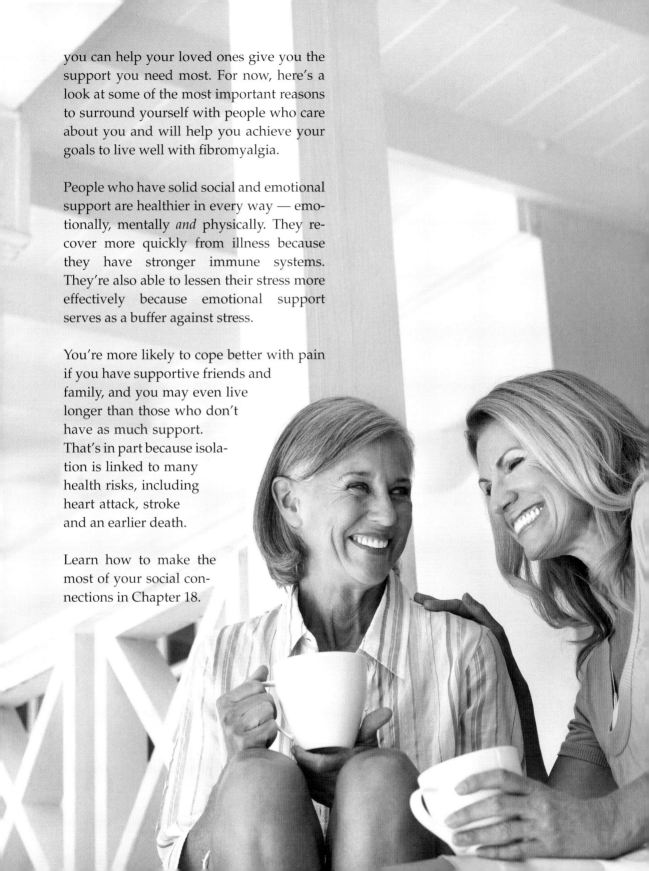

you can help your loved ones give you the support you need most. For now, here's a look at some of the most important reasons to surround yourself with people who care about you and will help you achieve your goals to live well with fibromyalgia.

People who have solid social and emotional support are healthier in every way — emotionally, mentally *and* physically. They recover more quickly from illness because they have stronger immune systems. They're also able to lessen their stress more effectively because emotional support serves as a buffer against stress.

You're more likely to cope better with pain if you have supportive friends and family, and you may even live longer than those who don't have as much support. That's in part because isolation is linked to many health risks, including heart attack, stroke and an earlier death.

Learn how to make the most of your social connections in Chapter 18.

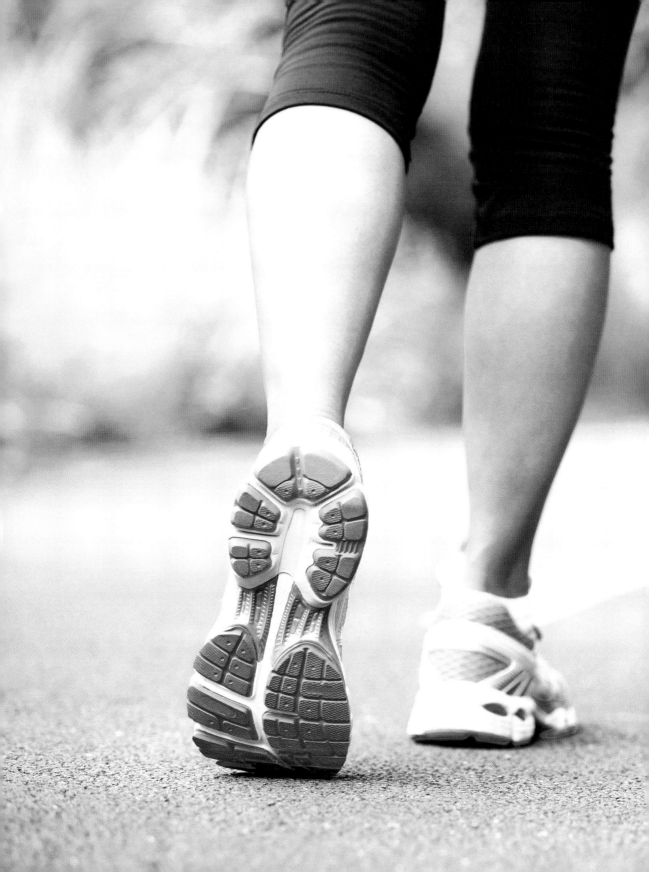

PART 4

Living with fibromyalgia

Whether you have fibromyalgia or have a loved one affected by it, this part of the book has something for everyone. The purpose of this section is to take what you've learned and put it into action.

In the first two chapters, you'll learn how to talk to your health care team and your loved ones. From there, you'll take what you've learned and condense it into a personal treatment plan. The pages that follow offer guidance to help you every step of the way. This personal plan is the key to getting your life back and moving forward, living your best life now — even with fibromyalgia.

Let's begin by visiting with Gloria and Justus, whom you first met in Chapter 1. Their success stories will set the stage for what you'll learn in the final part of this book.

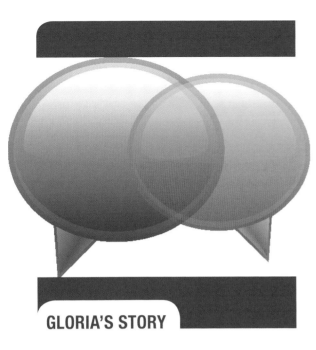

GLORIA'S STORY

'Never give up'

When Gloria was first told that she had fibromyalgia, she didn't believe it. Her health history was riddled with many different medical conditions, and any one (or combination) could be to blame for how she was feeling.

"I just kind of stored it up there in my little box of unexplained things and thought, *Well, we'll see how this plays out,*" Gloria said. "It really took a while for me to sort it out because I was dealing with so many health issues."

Gloria was left with a diagnosis of fibromyalgia but not much of a plan for what to do about it. And so began her journey to where she is today. Through it all, Gloria has learned to never give up.

Lessons to learn

Loss was the first lesson fibromyalgia taught Gloria. Gloria and her husband had been serving in a ministry for a couple of years. Although things had been going well, as time passed, Gloria's symptoms left her feeling that she didn't have enough energy to keep the ministry going, so she and her husband chose to shut it down.

"I think I cried for a year," Gloria said. "I was just so distraught over not being able to fulfill that calling in my life."

And then there were Gloria's hobbies: sewing, knitting and crocheting. "I just can't do them anymore," Gloria said.

She also took pride in keeping an immaculate house. "I was a neat freak. I had to have everything ordered." That changed, too.

One by one, the losses Gloria experienced changed her life. "It was a grief process I had to go through," she recalls.

Making lemonade out of limitations

Gloria still struggles with limitations today, but through her struggles, she has learned how to find joy and fulfillment even with the changes that fibromyalgia has brought into her life.

One of the first things Gloria learned that helped her move forward was accepting that her situation wasn't going to change.

SECRETS TO GLORIA'S SUCCESS

When Gloria thinks about the strategies that help her cope with fibromyalgia, it's not hard for her to put together a list of what works for her. Here are her tips:

- Keep your sense of humor. Laugh a lot.
- Be willing to rethink the expectations you have for yourself. Sometimes your expectations have to change and you have to feel that loss — and then seek out new opportunities.
- Don't get easily offended by others. Not everyone will understand what you're experiencing with fibromyalgia.
- Stay flexible. If you're not flexible, Gloria says, you'll break. "You've got to be willing to change and allow changes around you, moment by moment," she says.
- Keep a positive attitude. Draw strength from somewhere that will help you keep going. For Gloria, her strength comes from her religious faith.
- Be grateful for each new day.
- Have faith in yourself and in your doctors.
- When you need to, "pick yourself up, dust yourself off and start all over again." Gloria is fond of these lyrics from a Frank Sinatra song.

"Keep going, moment by moment," Gloria says. "No matter how difficult the road ahead appears to be, never give up."

"It's how to perceive it and deal with it that's going to change," she said. "You're going to have to make changes if you want to live some sort of a balanced life."

Gloria no longer grieves for what she used to do. Instead, she accepts who she is and what she's able to do today. There are times when that acceptance doesn't come easily, but Gloria's goal is to continue to live life to the fullest in the ways that she can.

"There are days or even periods of days where fibromyalgia just takes over my life completely," Gloria says. "I have learned over the years, though, what that process is like, and if I know that I'm going into a crisis or difficult day, then I just refocus what I'm doing and take time to rest in different ways."

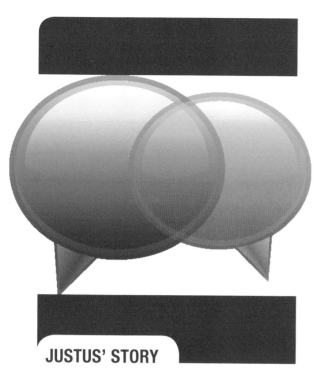

JUSTUS' STORY

'I'm thankful'

Ask Justus Wilder what he did after he found out he had fibromyalgia, and he won't hesitate to tell you that he suffered for 11 long months. He suffered because he couldn't figure out on his own how to feel better.

"It was just a really bad spot, and I had to come to the realization that this was going to be fixed, and this was going to be fixed by me," Justus said. With that thought in mind, Justus signed up for a three-week pain rehabilitation program.

In the program, Justus learned about the strategies that you've been reading about in this book. They're designed to help people manage their symptoms and live enjoyable, fulfilling lives with fibromyalgia. He uses the same daily planner you'll complete for yourself later in this book.

Today, Justus is no longer suffering. Instead, he's thankful.

"I'm not thankful that I have it, but since I have it, I'm thankful," Justus says about fibromyalgia. "It took me a while to get to this point, and it wasn't easy at all. But the fact is, [fibromyalgia is] part of me. It's a part of my routine now, how I live my life. In no way, shape or form do I wish that I *didn't* have it, because it has made me better. It has made me more aware of life."

Sticking to the plan

Justus doesn't claim to have a perfect quality of life all the time — he has good and bad days just like everyone else. But he says that his life is better on the days when he sticks to the daily plan he sets for himself. That means waking up and going to bed at the same time every day, taking breaks, not overdoing it, and making sure not to cut himself off from others — especially on his bad days.

"When those things line up, my quality of life is better than it was," Justus says. "Nobody's going to have a perfect weekly schedule. But if I can throw time in there for myself and if I really stick to the waking up and going to sleep at the same time, my quality of life tends to be pretty good."

SECRETS TO JUSTUS' SUCCESS

Among the top strategies Justus uses to manage his fibromyalgia, he:

- *Stretches daily.* Justus tries to do all of the stretches you'll find in this book (see page 242) every day. "Stretching is the biggest thing," Justus says. "I can feel if I don't stretch in the morning. I can't go without those stretches." He says it's a night-and-day difference on the days that he stretches versus the days that he doesn't.
- *Takes breaks.* He applies the 20-20-20 rule: Every 20 minutes he spends looking at a computer, he looks at something 20 feet away for 20 seconds. This has been especially helpful for him on days when he has to use a computer a lot. "If I don't, and I continuously stare at that computer screen, my day goes downhill. My eyes start to get watery and heavy and my head starts to hurt," Justus says. "The pain starts to rev up, and everything just falls to the wayside."
- *Sticks to his daily schedule.* And for Justus, this means giving his schedule some breathing room. "I don't fill my whole calendar up. Not overloading that schedule is helpful," Justus says. His calendar plots his day out in 30-minute increments, and he tries to keep some slots open so he doesn't overload his schedule. At the same time, those open blocks of time give him flexibility for the times when something unexpected comes up.
- *Gets daily exercise.* For an hour or two after work, you'll find Justus doing cardio, lifting weights, using exercise bands and even boxing for a little extra cardio.
- *Takes time for himself.* "Taking time for myself during the day has really helped me," Justus says. "We live in a fast world with fast cars and fast things going on, always having to do something and go somewhere, and I'm the worst at it. I find that taking a minute and sitting back and taking a breath and taking time for yourself, whether it's a 10-minute bubble bath or a 10-minute walk around the park or whatever you need to do."
- *Reads or listens to something relaxing* for 30 minutes before going to sleep.
- *Tries to keep life in perspective.* "If you can get to a place where (you can tell yourself), 'Hey, I'm in a better position than most people.' If you can get to that point, I think that makes things easier."

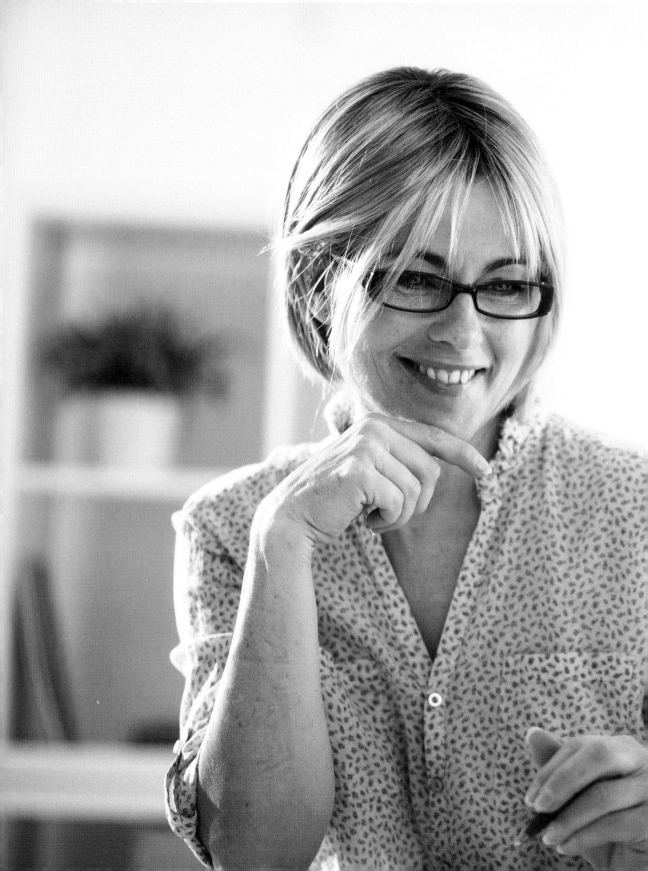

CHAPTER 17

Partnering with your doctor

Chances are that you've traveled down a long and bumpy road to get to this point. For many people with fibromyalgia, a true diagnosis can take years and involve several medical tests and doctors, not to mention a fair share of frustration and heartache. It can be an enormous relief to finally get validation from a medical professional that your pain and other symptoms aren't in your head — they're real, and they're caused by a known condition.

The flip side of that relief is learning that you have a condition that doesn't currently have a cure. That means you'll have to manage it like other chronic illnesses, such as diabetes or high blood pressure.

There's good news in this. Although there isn't a cure for fibromyalgia, it can be successfully managed. The goal of this book is to help you enjoy the best quality of life possible, even with fibromyalgia. The tools and strategies you've read about in this book have helped many people with fibromyalgia manage their symptoms and live fulfilling, enjoyable lives. That means they can help you, too.

While managing fibromyalgia largely rests in your hands, your health care team can offer invaluable guidance and support along the way.

The pages that follow offer tips and suggestions to help you make the most of your partnership with your health care team.

"TODAY, MORE DOCTORS THAN EVER HAVE A BETTER GRASP OF THE CONDITION."

AN EVOLVING UNDERSTANDING

Since the American College of Rheumatology put fibromyalgia on the map in 1990, it has been recognized as one of the most common chronic pain conditions. A growing body of research has helped people learn more about the causes of fibromyalgia and the most helpful treatments. Today, more doctors than ever have a better grasp of the condition. And the learning continues.

With that said, people with fibromyalgia can bump up against a knowledge gap when it comes to their own doctor. Not all doctors are on the front lines of fibromyalgia research; that means they're not always aware of the latest information about the condition. Some doctors may even be a bit skeptical about the disorder in general. This can make treating the condition frustrating for both you and your doctor.

Whether your health care team knows a lot or very little about fibromyalgia, keep in mind that they want to help you, even if they haven't been able to in the past. With the information in this book, you're gathering the knowledge and tools you need to take charge of your health and build a positive partnership with your health care team.

WHO SHOULD GUIDE YOUR CARE?

One of your first steps is to decide who to work with to manage your symptoms. Many people with fibromyalgia receive their diagnosis from a rheumatologist. This is a doctor who focuses on arthritis and other similar conditions. A rheumatologist will help rule out other problems first and then officially diagnose your fibromyalgia. Once this step has taken place, who should guide your care?

After a diagnosis, the best person to lead your care is a trusted primary care doctor or another primary care provider who knows your health history. This should be someone you're comfortable with; someone who can work with you to meet your health care needs. This person serves as your first point of contact for ongoing and new health concerns alike.

Think of your doctor as your team coach. He or she can help you devise your game plan, refer you to other health care providers as needed, and coordinate all the members of your health care team.

Now that you know who should coach your team, what's your role? You're the star quar-

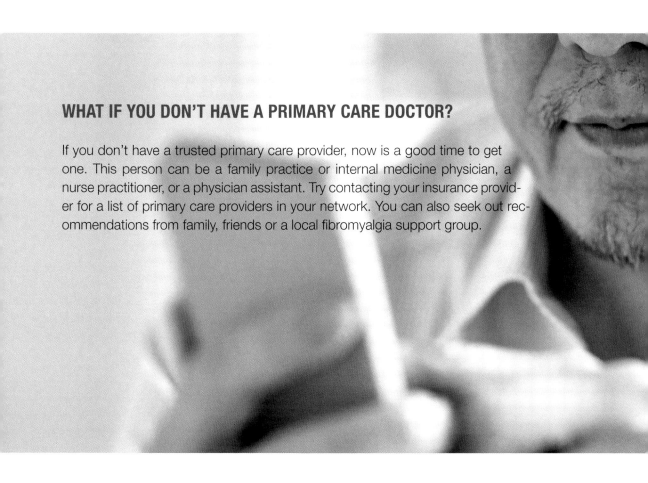

WHAT IF YOU DON'T HAVE A PRIMARY CARE DOCTOR?

If you don't have a trusted primary care provider, now is a good time to get one. This person can be a family practice or internal medicine physician, a nurse practitioner, or a physician assistant. Try contacting your insurance provider for a list of primary care providers in your network. You can also seek out recommendations from family, friends or a local fibromyalgia support group.

terback. It's up to you to carry out the game plan and get the ball down the field. While your doctor can help you get there, the fact is that he or she can't do your treatment plan for you.

Building a partnership

When your symptoms first appeared, you probably were hoping for a quick diagnosis and an easy fix. When this didn't happen, you and your doctor likely both felt frustrated and disappointed.

Now that you have a diagnosis, the best way to get the most out of working with your health care team is to build a partnership with your doctor.

To do that, it helps to first have a realistic idea of what you would like to see happen going forward. Try thinking of your doctor as someone you'll work with, rather than someone who can "fix" how you're feeling. This change in thinking will empower you to take charge of your health care and your treatment plan. It will allow you to seek guidance and support rather than a cure.

And it can open up new opportunities for you and your doctor to tackle your symptoms together.

Equally helpful is the understanding that you're gaining just by reading this book. Page by page, you're learning about what fibromyalgia is, as well as the most effective ways to manage it. When you approach your doctor not only with a diagnosis but with the ability to take control of your health care, he or she will be better able to help you put your treatment plan into action.

Seeing your relationship with your doctor as a partnership offers other benefits, too:

Better communication. A true partnership between you and your doctor leads to better communication. Better communication can create a more satisfying experience with your doctor and cut down on frustration as you learn how to manage your symptoms.

Lower risk of overmedication. When you're able to talk to and work well with your doctor, you're better able to make and stick to a daily treatment plan that will help you manage your symptoms. This can make it less likely that you'll be overprescribed medications that aren't helpful for treating fibromyalgia symptoms.

Improved symptoms. Research has shown that people with fibromyalgia who partner well with their doctor are more committed to their treatment plan. That kind of commitment leads to better overall health in people with chronic conditions.

Making the most of your office visit

Some people with fibromyalgia see their doctor once or twice a year. Others schedule visits more regularly. When and how often you see your doctor is up to the two of you. Either way, it's a good idea to have a plan for your appointments so that you can get the most out of your time together.

Here are some ideas to keep in mind before your next office visit:

Bring your list of medications. Keep an up-to-date list of any medications you're currently taking. Be sure to include supplements on your list, too.

Keep a list of questions. Divide any questions you have for your doctor into urgent and not-so-urgent concerns. That way, you can be sure to get to the most pressing questions first.

Have a plan in hand. Whether you want to start a new exercise routine, improve your diet or work toward getting better sleep, let your doctor know what you plan to try. This way, you'll be sure that your plan is a good fit for your situation. If needed, your doctor can then give you tips for putting your plan into action.

Focus on one or two specific goals. Some people find that it's helpful to tackle one or two symptoms at a time. For example, you may want to focus the appointment on lessening your pain, addressing your fatigue or improving the quality of your sleep.

Talk about your exercise plan. This is especially important if you haven't been exercising much before now or if you have other health conditions that may affect your ability to exercise. Your doctor can help you decide on an exercise plan that will be safe and effective for you.

Ask about physical therapy. Your doctor can help you decide if you'd benefit from this type of support.

Raise any concerns about mood or depression. If you're struggling with depression, be sure to bring it up with your doctor. He or she can help you come up with a plan that may include counseling, medication or another therapy.

Leave with a shared understanding of your treatment plan. Before your appointment ends, make sure you're both on the same page. Taking notes during your appointment or bringing a family member or trusted friend with you may be helpful.

Commit to the plan. Make a commitment to follow the treatment that you and your doctor decide is best. Then at your next appointment, you can report back on how it's gone and share any adjustments or additions you've made.

Responsibility and partnership go hand in hand

By taking responsibility for your health and fully engaging in your treatment plan, you're in a better position to build a successful partnership with your doctor. By working together with your doctor and others on your health care team, you can manage your symptoms, stay committed to your treatment plan, and improve your overall health and quality of life.

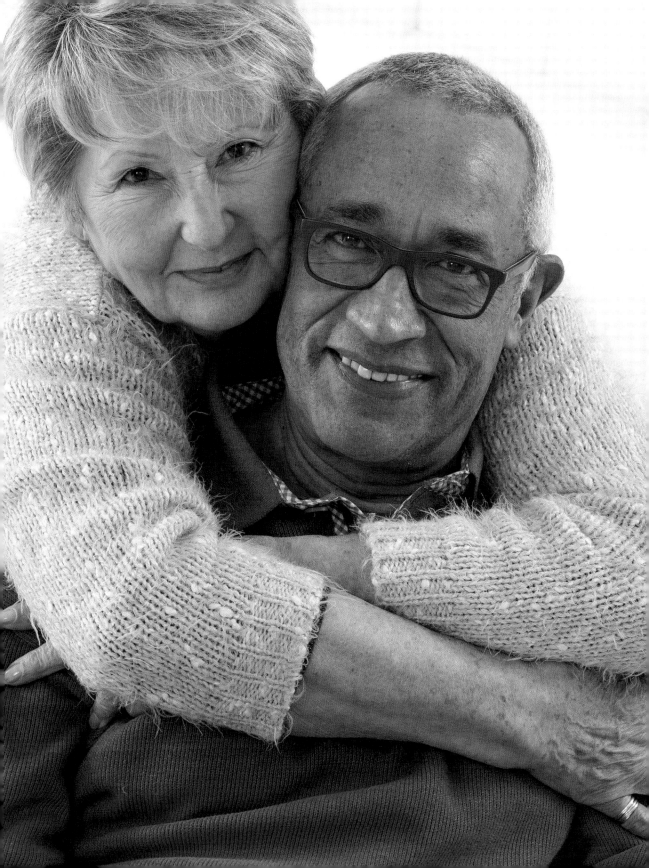

CHAPTER 18

Family and support

Many people with fibromyalgia struggle to open up about the extent of their pain and the sense of loss they may be feeling. If you've always been an independent, take-charge kind of person, reaching out for a helping hand can be uncomfortable and even frightening. You may worry that you'll become a burden to your loved ones if you ask for and accept their help. You may fear that you'll lose your sense of identity and role in the family or be seen as weak.

Even if you're comfortable with seeking support, ongoing symptoms such as pain and fatigue can affect how much you want to engage with others. When you're having a bad day, the last thing you may feel like doing is spending time with family or taking a walk with a friend. Then, without realizing it, you may find that you've isolated yourself from the people you care about.

Yet the support of your family and friends is more important now than ever. By letting your loved ones in, you'll be better equipped to take control of your fibromyalgia symptoms and lead a fuller, more satisfying life.

WHY SUPPORT MATTERS

Looking to others for support is one of the best ways you can get a leg up on fibromyalgia. Research has shown again and again that those who get positive support from the people in their lives are better able to cope with chronic conditions such as fibromyalgia. Here's how a strong support network can help.

Greater acceptance

People with chronic disorders say that friends and family have played a central role in helping them come to terms with their condition and move forward in their lives. Your support system can help you dwell less on what you've lost and focus more on strategies to start feeling better.

Added self-confidence

A strong support system has been shown to boost people's confidence in their ability to handle the ups and downs of a chronic condition. In turn, this self-assuredness makes it more likely that you'll be able to manage your condition successfully and boost your quality of life.

Improved symptoms

The support of family and friends may improve how you feel day to day.

In one study, women with good support systems were less sensitive to fibromyalgia pain. These women felt that their condition had less of an impact on their daily lives. They also felt that they were better able to function. Research also suggests that chronic pain improves in the long term for people who regularly receive empathy from a close loved one, such as a spouse.

Better motivation

As you've already learned, managing fibromyalgia largely rests in your hands. When you find something that improves your symptoms — whether it's daily exercise, better nutrition or meditation — one of the best things you can do is to stick with it. Your support system can be instrumental in keeping you motivated. Many studies have shown that when people with chronic conditions have the support of family and friends, they remain more committed to their self-treatment plans.

A more positive attitude

Research shows that a strong social network is linked to a more positive outlook on life and better mood in people with fibromyalgia. Studies also suggest that support from family and friends leads to better mental health and stronger ability to handle stress.

Increased happiness and well-being

People who have positive social support in their lives are shown to be happier and feel better about life overall. Spending time with loved ones and sharing positive experiences together can take your mind off your symptoms and boost your mood. Connecting with family and friends can also increase your sense of belonging and purpose, both of which help boost overall well-being.

HELPING YOUR FAMILY HELP YOU

If you're like many people with fibromyalgia, you may find it daunting to talk openly about your condition. Where do you start? How do you get others to understand something they can't see? You may feel that no matter how supportive others are, they'll never understand fibromyalgia without experiencing it themselves. Rather than repeatedly explaining what you're going through, it may seem easier to withdraw and keep your pain to yourself.

Despite these challenges, you owe it to your family and yourself to bring them into the loop. The more they know about fibromyalgia, the better they'll be able to support you.

If your loved ones are kept in the dark, they may feel confused about your health and struggle to find the best way to help. Their worries and fears may magnify if they think certain things about what's going on inside your body that aren't true — all because they don't understand.

As the saying goes, "Knowledge is power." By teaching your family about what fibromyalgia is and isn't, you'll be empowering them to become a positive source of support. A good place to start might be Chapter 3 in this book, which outlines common myths and facts about fibromyalgia.

Whether you're just breaking the news to your family or wanting to open up more with them, here are some tips that can help you effectively talk about fibromyalgia with your loved ones.

Have a plan

If you're sharing your diagnosis with family members, you may want to think through what you're going to say first. It may be helpful to write a list of the details you want to share and tailor that list for different friends and family members.

For example, you'll likely go into more depth with a spouse or partner than you will with a young child. Or you may know that your mother will be reassured by as many details as you can offer. Your sister, on the other hand, might be overwhelmed by a flood of information.

Start with the facts

Explain what fibromyalgia is in a simple, straightforward way. Don't get too caught up in theories at this point. Stick to what's known about the condition. Here are some key pieces of information you might share:
- Fibromyalgia is a chronic disorder. The most common symptoms are widespread pain and fatigue. Other common signs and symptoms include problems with sleep, memory and mood.
- There's no cure for fibromyalgia, but symptoms can get better.

Describe your treatment plan

Let your family know what steps you're taking to improve your symptoms and live as full a life as possible. Tell them, for example, that your symptoms improve when you exercise regularly, reduce stress and get a full night's sleep. The more they know, the better they can support you in your self-treatment plan. Later in this book (see page 236), you'll create a personal plan that you'll use every day. You may find it helpful to share this plan with your loved ones.

Invite your spouse or partner to your doctor's appointments

By hearing what you and your doctor discuss, your loved one may gain a deeper insight into what you're going through. This, in turn, can help your loved one understand what he or she can do to help.

As a bonus, having someone else with you in the room can also help you in a number of other ways. A loved one can help make sure that all of your questions are answered and that you remember to ask questions that you wanted to bring up. A loved one can also help you after the appointment if you happen to forget something that your doctor said.

Offer additional sources of information

Encourage your family to learn about fibromyalgia. Point them in the direction of good sources of information that explain more about the condition and how family members can help. The chapter of additional resources at the end of this book may be a good starting point.

Define common medical terms

Depending on your symptoms, some terms are likely to come up on a regular basis. It may be helpful for your family to become familiar with terms such as *fibro fog, irritable bowel syndrome (IBS)* or *interstitial cystitis.* The glossary in this book may help.

Explain that you need to take things as they come

Fibromyalgia is unpredictable — this is an important point to make. That can make it hard sometimes to stick to rigid routines or plans. You may need to do things a little differently so that you have the energy you need each day and can keep your symptoms under control. Revisit moderation and pacing in Chapter 14 and share tips with your loved ones if you think it might be helpful.

Expect some skeptics

You may find that some relatives seem to doubt what you're telling them or question you outright. Try giving them helpful sources of information (see page 256) or inviting them to accompany you to a doctor's appointment to learn more.

COMMUNICATION DO'S AND DON'TS

When you talk to your loved ones about your fibromyalgia, use these additional tips to help guide your conversations.

DO	DON'T
Share what you're going through. Don't isolate yourself when you're having a bad day or bottle up your grief, sadness or worries. Talking can relieve strain and help you see the bigger picture. It may lead to a healthy plan of action.	**Complain all the time.** Sometimes, people rely too heavily on behaviors, such as groaning and wincing, to get care and support from others. This makes your symptoms more of a focus than the healthy parts of your life. Too much complaining can also push people away.
Be assertive. Assertive communication means sharing your needs, feelings and ideas in an open, honest and direct way. It promotes mutual respect and problem-solving.	**Be aggressive.** Aggressive communication blames, hurts and often offends other people or puts them down. When you speak aggressively, other people become defensive and relationship problems often happen.
Encourage openness. Allow your loved ones to ask questions and talk through any confusion, frustration or fears they're having. Be patient with them and keep the lines of communication open.	**Dismiss your family's thoughts and feelings.** Don't brush aside their questions or concerns as unimportant. Try to put yourself in their shoes and understand where they're coming from.
Be aware of your family's needs. Take an interest in your loved ones' lives by asking questions and being a good listener. Encourage them to take care of their own health and well-being.	**Assume you're the only one who needs support.** Your relationship with your family will be stronger — and you'll work better together as a team — if your loved ones know you're supporting them as much as they're supporting you.

If all else fails, you may have to accept that some people have a hard time changing their mindsets. In those cases, it's OK to protect yourself by limiting the time you spend with negative or critical people.

Seek professional help

If you find it hard to talk to your loved ones, a therapist or another member of your health care team may be able to help.

BUILD YOUR TEAM OF SUPPORT

Some people with fibromyalgia have supportive families that rally quickly to their side. Others don't.

Whatever your situation, it's a good idea to expand your support system beyond family members. Research shows that people with a diverse support system that includes friends, family and health care providers cope better with chronic conditions and enjoy better health and well-being.

Try making a list of people you can reach out to. As you create your list, don't limit it to the most obvious people. You might be surprised by who ends up being a helpful source of support — maybe it's a neighbor who's striving to take daily walks or an empathetic co-worker who has chronic arthritis.

Local and online support groups for people with fibromyalgia can also be great resources. It can be deeply comforting to connect with and get advice from people who know what you're going through.

Keep in mind, though, that support groups can have their pitfalls. Beware of support groups that promise a cure for fibromyalgia, serve largely as a place for people to complain, have a leader who urges you to stop treatment, or are judgmental of your decisions or actions. An unhealthy support group is likely to do more harm than it does good.

The same goes for online support groups — and in those cases, it's also important to take care with how much personal information you share.

Here are additional suggestions to help you maintain or improve your support system.

Stay in touch. Attend family gatherings. Answer phone calls and respond to mail and email. Accept invitations to activities, even if it's hard to at first.

Take charge. Don't wait for someone else to make the first move. If you meet a potential good friend, invite him or her for coffee. Strike up a conversation while in line at the grocery store.

Accept every social invitation you receive. No matter how you feel, say yes to every single one. This means you are saying yes to your life again and regaining the activities and relationships that matter to you. This comes with one important caveat: Stay for only 30 minutes. While the key here is to participate in life, don't overdo it. As you build strength and stamina, you can increase how much time you spend on social activities.

Explore new options. Take part in community organizations, volunteer work and neighborhood events. Join a health club or hobby group or take a class.

Go on a date night every Saturday night. No matter how you're feeling, go out with your spouse or partner or someone else who cares about you — an adult child, a brother or sister, or a friend. Those closest to you are the ones who are best able to support you

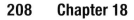

because they know about your life. Spending time with them increases that support. On your date night, get dressed, leave the house and above all, don't talk about your health.

Don't give up on existing relationships. Good relationships require patience, compromise and acceptance.

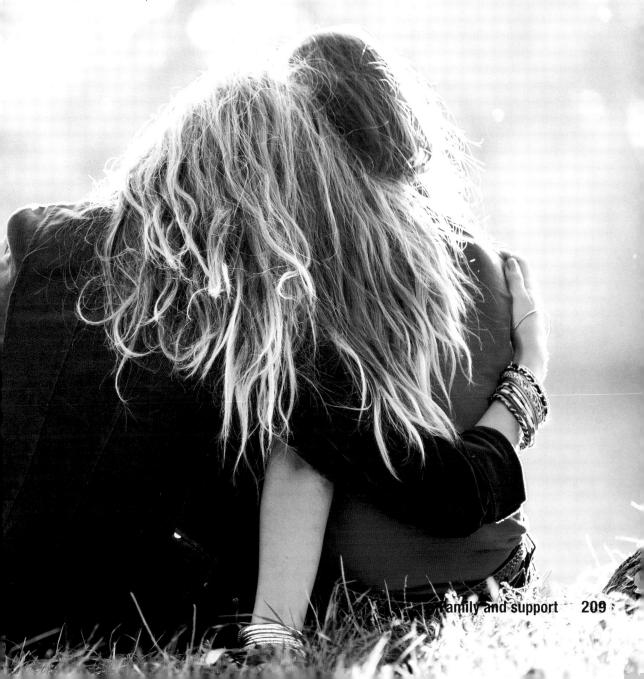

An outside expert may be able to offer suggestions on ways you can open communication channels.

HOW YOUR FAMILY CAN SUPPORT YOU

For people living with fibromyalgia, family can play a major role in managing the condition from day to day. Loved ones often get involved with decisions about care and may want to help you stay on track with your treatment plan. They can support healthy changes in sleep, exercise and eating habits, and provide helpful feedback to your health care team during appointments.

Just as valuable, family members can offer loving support by listening and expressing empathy, affection and care — and cheering you on as you take steps to manage your symptoms effectively.

These supportive efforts tend to fall into two categories: emotional and practical. If you're missing your daughter who left for college and someone offers you a compassionate listening ear, that's *emotional support*. If you're trying to exercise more and a loved one agrees to walk with you every evening after dinner, that's *practical support*.

Some people are good at giving both kinds of support, but you'll find that many people in your life are better at one or the other — and that's OK. Different members of your family can play different roles. If you expect one person to meet all your needs, you risk feeling disappointed or stretching that person too thin.

The important thing is to figure out what specific kinds of support would be most helpful to you — and then ask for it. Don't be afraid to speak up. Many families welcome the chance to get involved rather than remain helpless on the sidelines.

If your loved ones are looking for specific roles they can play in your life, consider sharing these suggestions.

Negotiate household roles and responsibilities

Work with your loved ones to create new routines at home. By redistributing certain chores and responsibilities, you'll be better able to pace yourself and limit physically painful tasks.

Just watch out for family members who want to do too much for you. Their hearts may be in the right place, but it's important that you play an active role in your life.

Stay informed

One of the best things your family can do is to learn about fibromyalgia. Suggest that your loved ones read up on the condition. There are many good sources of information on fibromyalgia — but there are plenty of unhelpful and even inaccurate sources out there, too.

Help ensure that they're finding the best information by pointing them toward the chapter of additional resources in this book (see page 256). Encourage them to come to your doctors' visits and attend fibromyalgia support group meetings with you.

From there, it's not your loved ones' duty to focus on your condition. Instead, your loved ones play an important role in helping you focus on truly living your life, whether it's a hobby, going to church, or any number of things that help ensure that you're truly living a meaningful and enjoyable life.

Support your exercise plan

Your family can motivate you to stay physically active by joining you in activities. Plan to go on regular walks together, meet for a weekly swim or sign up for a yoga class. (Learn more about physical activity in Chapter 13.)

Support good nutrition

If you're changing your eating habits as part of your self-management plan, family members can help you stick with those new habits. They can help with grocery shopping or pitch in with meal prep.

Together, you and your family can also agree to keep certain foods out of the house or store them in an out-of-the-way drawer or cabinet. (Learn more about the importance of nutrition starting on page 183.)

Help achieve better sleep

Getting enough sleep is an important part of coping with fibromyalgia, but good sleep can be elusive. Your family can help by supporting your efforts to stick to a regular bedtime schedule and pre-bedtime routine. (Learn more starting on page 175.)

Help reduce stress

Stress is a normal part of life, but too much stress can make your symptoms worse. Talk to your family about situations that trigger stress for you, and work together to limit or avoid those situations. For example, if loud, busy restaurants agitate you, agree to eat out before or after the dinner crowd. Or if a packed weekend schedule feels overwhelming, work together to build in periods of rest. Family members can also encourage you to practice relaxation techniques and join you in activities, such as meditation or tai chi. (Learn more about managing stress starting on page 164.)

Support efforts to use your energy wisely

Moderation and pacing are two important tools that will help ensure that you have the energy you need to live a full, enjoyable and productive life. Understanding how moderation and pacing work (see Chapter 14) can help your loved ones respect and support your efforts to use your energy well on a day-to-day basis.

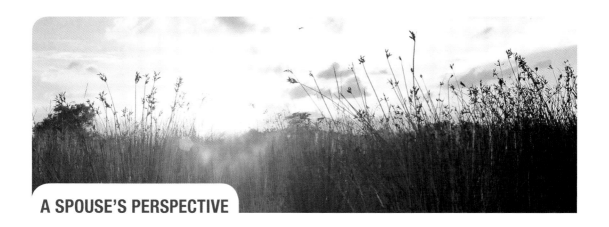

A SPOUSE'S PERSPECTIVE

Mike reflects on his wife's fibromyalgia

Editor's note: Earlier in this book (see pages 16 and 192), you read about Gloria's experience with fibromyalgia. What follows is Gloria's husband's perspective on the condition.

Mike and Gloria started out as partners in a high school square-dancing class. Today, after more than 50 years of marriage, they're still partners in every sense of the word. It's that sense of commitment that's helped them weather life's ups and downs — including those with fibromyalgia.

Mike describes Gloria as very energetic in the early days of their courtship. She was involved with Girl Scouts, water-skied and contributed to a local newspaper, all while getting good grades in school. Gloria carried this energy and ambition into her adult and family life after she and Mike were married.

"(She was) very energetic, very involved with everything, kept a spectacular house, cooked, cleaned — she did all of that while she was pregnant," Mike said. To add to this, Mike was in the Navy, so they were apart during his deployments. This meant that Gloria sometimes had to keep everything together — maintaining their house and raising their two children — on her own.

Once they were together for good, life for Mike and Gloria didn't skip a beat. "She worked a job during the day; I worked nights," Mike said. "Anything that we wanted to do with our families, picnics or that sort of stuff, was never a concern. We just did it. There was one time when we had only one car and our washer and dryer went on the fritz, so she would put the kids in the carriage and push them about a half a mile and go to a laundromat. There was never any hesitation. She was a Cub Scout leader, a Sunday school teacher … she just did it."

Then one day, things started to change. The changes weren't instant, and they didn't happen overnight. But something was happening to the Gloria that Mike had known and loved for so many years.

Mysterious symptoms

"I'd seen this lady be unstoppable to then all of a sudden almost unmovable. She'd have to lay down and take a nap," Mike said.

Gloria's symptoms were puzzling for Mike, who describes himself as a "black-and-white person." "There's a cause and an effect," Mike said. "You hit your finger with a hammer, and it's going to hurt. I learned that that's not always the case."

Doctor after doctor couldn't pinpoint a cause for Gloria's symptoms. To make things worse, few people understood what Gloria was going through because she didn't look any different. "There are a lot of people who look at a person and they say, 'Well, you look good. You've got to be hitting on all eight cylinders,'" Mike said. "(But) a lot of people don't recognize that you might look OK, but you can be hurting inside." Such was the case with Gloria, and Mike knew it.

Confusion over what was causing Gloria's symptoms eventually led to anger for Mike. *Why can't somebody help?* he wondered.

But through it all, Mike believed in Gloria. "We just rolled up our sleeves and kept on truckin'," Mike says of the journey it took to find an answer to Gloria's symptoms. Then in 2001, they learned Gloria had fibromyalgia.

"It wasn't a eureka, like oh, God, now we have a name; OK, now you're not going to have these problems anymore — that's not the case," Mike says of his reaction to the news that Gloria had fibromyalgia. "But I think it was maybe a little bit reassuring that they have a name and there's this medical team that's working on this specifically."

'Flexible with a capital F'

As they set out to learn everything they could about fibromyalgia, Mike and Gloria learned another word that started with an F that would become a part of their daily vocabulary: flexibility. "You just learn to be flexible with a capital F," Mike says. "We joke around here that if you're not flexible, you'll break. You roll with it the best you can."

Rolling with it meant understanding when Gloria needed to rest or to do things differently than she had before. On days when Gloria's feeling more sensitive to noise, for example, they choose to go to a quieter restaurant. For Mike, managing fibromyalgia — and in this case, helping his wife cope with her symptoms — has meant day-to-day and, sometimes, moment-to-moment choices.

Another word, this time starting with a capital C, has taken on a starring role in Mike's life as he continues to support his wife's efforts in managing fibromyalgia.

"You should be very considerate, with a capital C," Mike says. "You have to be considerate and patient. You can't be combative. Be understanding, patient and considerate."

"We're in this together, she and I. Whatever we have to do, we're going to do."

DO'S AND DON'TS FOR FAMILY MEMBERS

Navigating life with a loved one who has fibromyalgia can be tricky. If you're in need of ways you can support a loved one who has fibromyalgia, these tips may help.

DO	DON'T
Think of the person with fibromyalgia as the expert. Your loved one understands his or her body and condition better than anyone else does. Your trust can help your loved one feel confident about managing this condition.	**Criticize or nag.** Avoid second-guessing or pestering. This may hamper your loved one's ability to effectively manage fibromyalgia symptoms. If you have genuine concerns, try to express them in a respectful way.
Ask how you can help. The kind of help your loved one needs may change as symptoms change. Ask what you can do to lend your support.	**Assume.** What you think might be helpful may actually be hurtful or stifling. Ask your loved what kind of support would be most helpful.
Be responsive. Be aware of what your loved one is going through and respond with the right kind of support. This is one way you can help your loved one reduce stress and feel better.	**Try to do it all.** In an attempt to be supportive, you may take over tasks that your loved one can do. This kind of overprotectiveness can backfire, causing your loved one to feel helpless.
Be positive. Take time to appreciate your loved one's strengths and abilities. Offer positive feedback when you see that your loved one is practicing healthy habits that help keep symptoms under control.	**Focus on the negative.** It's easier for your loved one to keep a positive attitude if you focus on the positive, too. A negative attitude about symptoms or limitations can come across as hurtful or judgmental.
Have fun together. Plan to do things you enjoy as a family several times a week. Sharing pleasurable experiences will bond you as a family and help get your mind off your loved one's pain.	**Forget to laugh.** Laughter can improve your mood, reduce stress and ease pain. Watch a comedy together, read jokes or recall humorous family memories.
Take care of yourself. Helping a loved one deal with chronic pain can take a toll on family members. It's OK to share how you feel and take time for yourself.	**Push your own needs aside.** If you put your loved one's needs before your own, you risk depleting your emotional and physical reserves.

WORK TOGETHER AS A TEAM

Loved ones are an invaluable resource when it comes to coping well with fibromyalgia. They can shore up your confidence, help you make important health decisions and support your efforts to improve how you feel. In turn, be sure to express your appreciation of them by being thankful and taking an active interest in their lives.

By working together, you can meet whatever challenges fibromyalgia may bring and continue to lead rich, satisfying lives.

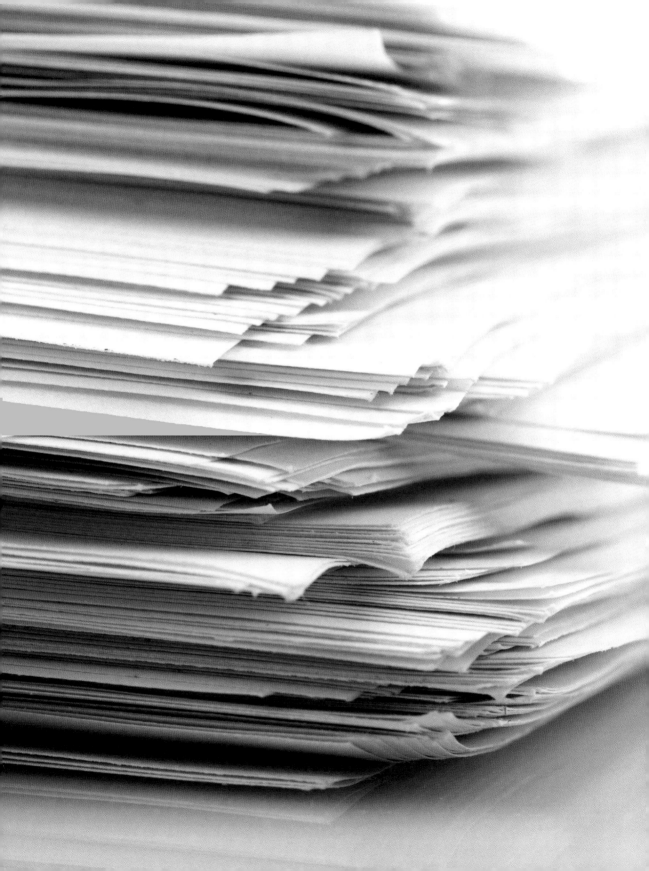

CHAPTER 19

Work life

As you likely already know, fibromyalgia can affect you in many ways from one day to the next. Pain, fogginess and other symptoms can make going to work feel like a struggle. You may even wonder if you might be better off not working at all.

You may feel that your symptoms make it difficult, if not impossible, to work. But there are many reasons to keep working. And there are many ways you can make your working life work for you. This chapter briefly outlines your options.

TO WORK OR NOT TO WORK?

You may feel as though fibromyalgia is robbing you of everything that brings you joy. And if you're like many people, a fulfilling work life is part of that joy. Will having fibromyalgia keep you from working?

Just the thought of not working may fill you with a sense of fear, dread and worry. First, there are the practical concerns. Work offers financial security and health benefits, which can help you stress less. Health benefits may also help give you better access to health care, which may help you manage your symptoms. Working less — or not at all — can significantly change all of these aspects of your life.

In addition, you may worry that if you don't work, you'll let your co-workers down, or

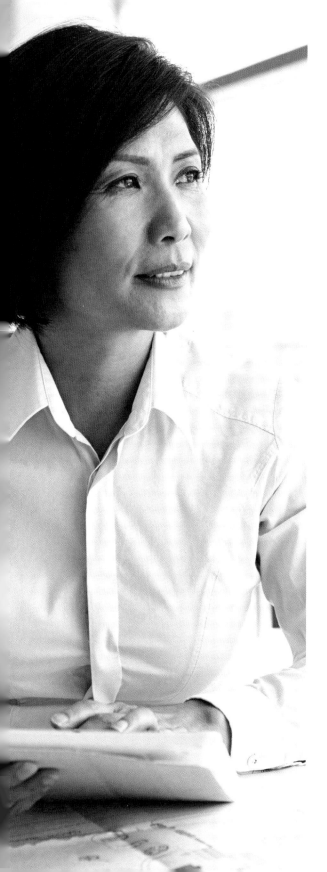

you'll disappoint your family because you won't be able to contribute in the ways that you always have. And then there's your personal sense of self-worth, purpose and identity — what will happen to them if you stop working?

At the same time, you may wonder if you can continue to work. Will the pain, fatigue and other symptoms you're feeling keep you from doing your best work? Or keep you from doing your job at all?

You may also wonder if more rest and less work-related stress would help you be a better parent or spouse. Put simply, would stepping away from work help you feel better? This swirl of thoughts can be frightening and overwhelming.

To work or not to work: This is a tough question to answer, and there's no one right answer for everyone with fibromyalgia. The choice you make is complex and individual. Although your loved ones and your health care team can help you decide which path to take, no one else can make this decision for you.

This chapter briefly addresses this difficult issue. An important part of this topic is how to pursue disability benefits if you decide not to work. Disability benefits are hard to obtain for people with fibromyalgia, as you'll learn.

Not working also leaves you with less income, which can present hardships on top of those you may already be facing.

THE AMERICANS WITH DISABILITIES ACT

The Americans with Disabilities Act (ADA) is a federal civil rights law that prevents job discrimination for people with certain disabilities. It applies to workplaces with 15 or more employees. The ADA protects people in areas such as hiring, firing, advancement, compensation and job training.

Specific medical conditions, such as fibromyalgia, aren't listed under the ADA. Instead, you must meet a general definition of disability. Under this definition, some people with fibromyalgia qualify as having a disability, while others do not.

Briefly, here's why. The most current definition of disability comes from the Americans with Disabilities Act Amendments Act of 2008. The term *disability* means a physical or mental impairment that substantially limits one or more major life activities, a record of such an impairment, or being regarded as having such an impairment. Major life activities include major bodily functions, such as digestion, thinking and breathing. Examples of life activities include performing manual tasks, seeing, hearing, lifting, reading, concentrating and communicating.

Some people with fibromyalgia may face many limitations in doing their work, while others may not be limited at all. Because there's such a variety of possible limitations and such a variety of different types of work, each person's situation needs to be considered individually to determine whether someone is unable to work because of the condition.

In appropriate situations, the ADA may require employers to make "reasonable accommodations" to help employees do their jobs. These may include allowing flexible work schedules and rest periods, reassigning some physically painful tasks to others, and making changes to an office space or work environment. Keep in mind that employers don't have to make changes that would cause them undue hardship, such as undertaking a significant expense. Workplaces also aren't required to make changes that could result in lower quality or production standards.

"WORKING MAY ALSO ALLOW BETTER HEALTH TO BE MAINTAINED OVER TIME."

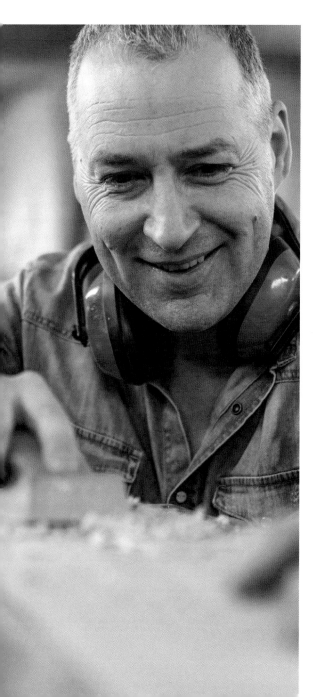

This chapter outlines your options, whether you choose to keep working or decide to pursue disability benefits.

WHAT RESEARCH SAYS

If you're facing the decision of whether to keep working or leave the workforce, you're already aware of some of the most important reasons to keep working. But what you may not know is that researchers have studied people with fibromyalgia and their work lives. These insights may help.

In general, research suggests that having a job may improve overall health and well-being for people with fibromyalgia. Working may also allow better health to be maintained over time.

People with fibromyalgia who work tend to feel less intense pain and fatigue and are less likely to feel depressed. They also have better physical and mental health, function better, and enjoy a higher quality of life.

Your job may also help you take the focus off your pain. It also provides your days with meaning and connects you to other people and the world around you.

Some people with fibromyalgia say that working helps them feel as though they're "beating" fibromyalgia rather than "giving in" to it. As one woman put it, "I will be crawling on the ground on my way to work before I give up and say, 'That's it, you win, fibromyalgia.'"

CAN FIBROMYALGIA BE DISABLING?

Although the reasons to stay at work are many, you may wonder if you should remain at your current job. Some people decide that their symptoms are affecting them so much that it's best to leave their jobs. This feeling varies from person to person and depends on many factors, such as the type of physical symptoms and how intense they are, mental health, the nature of the work, and the quality of workplace support.

Fibromyalgia has been viewed as a *potentially* disabling condition by the Social Security Administration since 2012. Of people who are diagnosed with fibromyalgia, as many as 1 in 3 leaves the workforce and receives disability benefits, either short term or long term. But many continue to work full time or part time.

What can make fibromyalgia disabling?

People who choose to stop working do so largely for these reasons.

Intensity of pain Severe pain is the No. 1 reason that a person with fibromyalgia stops working. The severity of other symptoms, such as fatigue and memory problems, also may be a factor.

Physical limitations People who are more limited in what they can do and how well they can function are more likely to stop working.

Job type Manual labor, repetitive movement or heavy lifting can be challenging for people with fibromyalgia. Individuals in physically demanding jobs are more likely to stop working, especially if they can't switch to a different job.

Lack of support and flexibility Research shows that support from others at work has a great impact on whether someone with fibromyalgia keeps working. It may be even more important than a person's pain. People who don't feel supported on the job may feel it's better not to work there at all.

DECIDING WHAT'S BEST FOR YOU

Before making any major decisions, talk to your health care team about your concerns. You may find that with certain lifestyle changes, such as getting more exercise or better sleep, you can continue to work.

It might also help to talk with your employer if you feel comfortable doing so. You may be able to flex your schedule, work part time rather than full time, avoid tasks that make your symptoms worse, or switch to a less stressful or strenuous position.

THE FAMILY MEDICAL LEAVE ACT

Some people request to take a temporary leave of absence from their jobs to focus on their health. The Family Medical Leave Act is a federal law that applies to employers with 50 or more employees. It requires that an employee with qualifying family or medical reasons be allowed to take unpaid leave for up to 12 weeks without losing his or her job.

One of those reasons includes "a serious health condition that makes the employee unable to perform the essential functions of his or her job." A leave of several weeks or months might be enough time for you to improve your symptoms so that you can continue working. For example, you may use this time for medical appointments and treatment.

Finally, talk to your family. Will you have the emotional and financial support you need to stop working? A financial adviser and close friends may be able to help you make your decision as well. If you do decide to pursue disability benefits and stop working, it's important to make sure you'll have the support of your loved ones.

Many people with fibromyalgia are able to keep working by making changes to their work situation and modifying how they perform their job duties. For example, you may build periods of rest into your day and schedule tasks around your daily patterns of high and low energy levels. In one study, a woman with fibromyalgia described her work life this way: "I might not do (the job) in the same way (my co-workers) would do it, but that doesn't mean I'm not going to get it done."

If, even with changes, you feel that where you work is no longer a good fit for you, you may seek a different job. Some people find less demanding positions in their fields. Others seek out educational or volunteer opportunities that allow them to retrain for jobs that are a better match.

All of these options lead back to the idea that working in some capacity, even if it's part time, may be a better choice than not working at all. Continuing to work helps you maintain your skills and stamina. Staying in the workforce in some form can also help keep isolation, loneliness and depression at bay.

APPLYING FOR DISABILITY BENEFITS

If you think that it's best to apply for disability benefits, talk to your doctor. If your doctor agrees, you'll
need to submit an application. The application process can take three to five months.

To qualify for disability benefits, your symptoms must be severe enough to meet
the government's definition of disability (see page 219). You must also prove that
your symptoms not only prevent you from doing the work you did in the past but
also impair you from doing any other type of skilled or unskilled work. Before you
start the application process, it can be helpful to take these steps.

Review your medical records. Ask for a copy of your medical records from all
the health care providers who have diagnosed or treated you. These records
should clearly document not only your diagnosis and office visits but also your
specific symptoms and limitations.

Keep your own records. For a brief period, keep a short, simple journal of your
day-to-day symptoms. Jot down how each symptom limits your ability to do
specific work-related tasks. Include details such as the intensity of the symptoms, how often they impair you and how long they last.

Work with your doctor. Share your personal records with your doctor. Ask that
your doctor add your personal information to your records if it isn't there already.

Consider meeting with a lawyer. If you can afford to, talk with a lawyer who
works on disability cases. A lawyer can tell you if you have a strong enough case
to successfully apply for disability benefits. You may also need a lawyer to make
an appeal if your first application is denied.

On average, more than three-quarters of all initial applications for disability benefits are denied. While you can go through several appeal processes with the
help of a lawyer, very few appeals result in approval for disability benefits.

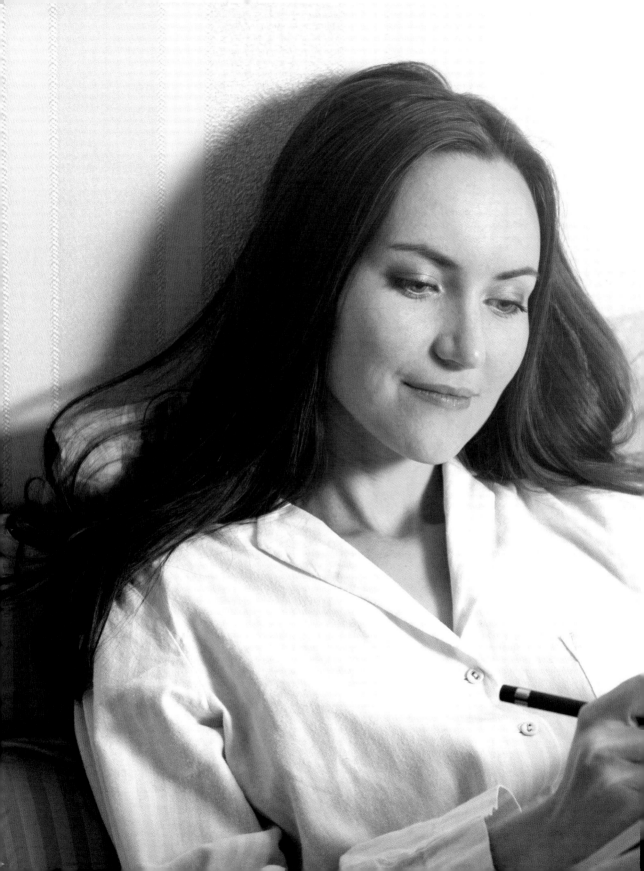

Action guide

This book has provided a lot of information about fibromyalgia. You've learned what it is and what it isn't. You've gained insight into its symptoms and its causes. You've gotten tips and advice to guide you as you manage your symptoms and talk to your health care team and your loved ones.

And if you're reading this book because someone you care about has fibromyalgia, you've gotten guidance on tools and strategies you can use to lend your support.

The next step is to put what you've learned into practice, and that's what you'll do in this chapter. This is where you'll develop a personal action guide that you can start using today. As you prepare to turn the page and start reading this chapter, get ready to start living your best life now.

CREATE YOUR PLAN

Now that you have a basic idea of what fibromyalgia is, it's time to take the next step: to start living your life more fully. Although there's no cure for fibromyalgia, you can manage this condition and live a meaningful, enjoyable life.

It's time to create your own personal plan for managing your symptoms and living better with fibromyalgia. At the end of this chapter, you'll find a daily planner that you can fill out and use every day. Fill out your planner with the guidance you receive as you read through this chapter.

Give your day structure

One of the first ways you can give your day structure is through your sleep habits. In addition to setting aside enough time for sleep, it's important to practice good sleep hygiene, as you learned in Chapter 16. One essential sleep habit that's important to adopt is going to bed and getting up at the same time every day.

Sleep is an important way to help relieve symptoms of fibromyalgia. It helps relieve fatigue, a common symptom. Sleep can also help reduce pain.

Experts have also found that the parts of your brain that regulate sleep may play a role in how fibromyalgia starts in the first place. These are the parts of the brain that are most affected by sleep disturbances.

Put simply, pairing a regular sleep cycle with good-quality sleep can help you manage fibromyalgia more effectively.

Plan it: On your daily planner (pages 236-237), write down what time you will go to bed and what time you will get up each day. Set a goal of 8½ hours — no more, no less.

Stretch your body – gently

Pain is the most common limiting factor of fibromyalgia. That makes stretching an important part of your daily plan. Gentle stretches can help you maintain function and carry out day-to-day activities. Perform gentle stretches first thing in the morning after you get up.

An added benefit of stretching is that it doesn't involve drugs, surgery, injections or physical therapy, and it doesn't cost anything. Stretching is considered a first-line treatment for relieving pain, helping reduce muscle spasms, and improving range of motion and function.

Combining stretching with strength training exercises can also help relieve pain. Learn more about strength training in Chapter 13. Find stretches to try starting on page 242 in the chapter of additional resources.

Plan it: On your daily planner (pages 236-237), write down when you'll do your stretches each day. Then, refer to the stretches starting on page 242 for step-by-step instructions.

ADJUSTING TO A NEW NORMAL

When change happens in life, it usually requires some sort of adjustment. Getting married, losing a parent or having a baby all are examples many people can relate to. The same is true with fibromyalgia. It's a change in your life that requires adjustment. Just as you can't go back to your life the way it was before you had a child, before your parent died or before you got married, it's not possible to go back to the way life was before fibromyalgia. Instead, it means adapting to a new normal.

It can be difficult to accept that you have fibromyalgia and move forward with your new normal. When you decide to take this step is completely up to you. Your doctor can help you figure out when you've seen enough specialists and had enough tests and are ready to move forward. Your doctor can also help you take all of the information you've learned and put it all together in a way that makes sense to you. Finally, your doctor can help you weigh the pros and cons of any remaining options you're considering.

Put simply, your doctor can help you sort through all of the information you have and decide when you're ready to move forward. From there, as you create your plan with the guidance in this chapter, your doctor and other members of your health care team can help answer any questions you have and provide support as you move forward.

Add movement to your day

Regular aerobic activity, in particular, has been shown to relieve pain, improve function and improve quality of life. But strengthening exercises can be helpful, too. Exercises that strengthen your muscles can help reduce pain and tenderness, improve how well you can carry out daily activities, and improve muscle strength and overall well-being.

You may also find symptom relief from water exercises (hydrotherapy). Water therapy has been shown to help relieve pain (learn more on page 140). It offers other benefits,

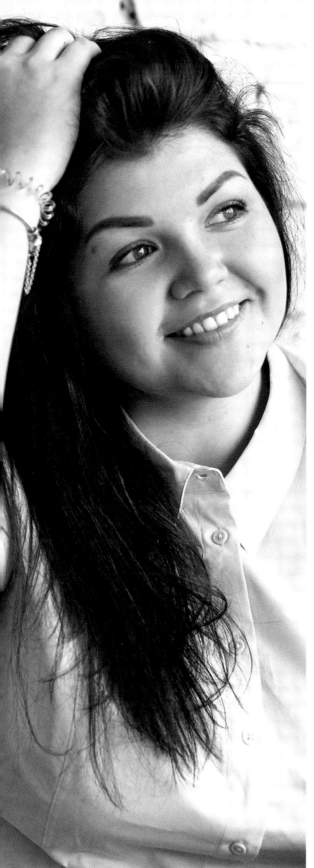

too. For example, it can improve your mood and how well you sleep. Warm water alone can even boost your confidence, helping you feel that getting regular physical activity is something you can achieve. With any exercise you do, keep your progress slow, gradual and steady.

Almost any physical activity is good for fibromyalgia. Use these three tips to help you choose activities and decide how much physical activity to get:
1. Choose activities that you enjoy.
2. Match the activities with your ability.
3. Pace yourself.

Set your physical activity goals so that you can meet them whether you're having a good day or a bad day. Walking, swimming, biking and water aerobics are all good low-impact choices. Yoga and tai chi are also good options (see page 108).

Plan it: Choose your physical activities and decide how long you'll do them and how many days a week you'll do them. Then add them to your planner (pages 236-237).

Keep stress in check

Living with fibromyalgia can be stressful. Stress, in turn, can worsen your symptoms. It's a vicious cycle. Stress can increase pain by causing you to tense your muscles, grit your teeth and stiffen your shoulders. In turn, as you feel more pain, you may feel less able to handle everyday tasks. This can lead to feeling frustrated, angry and depressed.

Your goal is to stop stress from snowballing and getting out of control. Take what you learned about stress management in Chapter 15 and put it into action.

Plan it: Choose stress-management techniques that you feel comfortable using every day. If you need ideas, revisit page 166. Then add the stress-management techniques you choose to your daily planner (pages 236-237).

Make time to relax

When you think about relaxation, maybe you think about things you enjoy doing in your spare time. Golfing, reading a good book or catching a movie are all examples.

While you may find these activities relaxing, they're actually examples of leisure. While leisure time is important, relaxation in this sense means exercises that help calm your body and your mind. These types of exercises have been shown to help people with fibromyalgia reduce their pain.

Plan it: Choose relaxation exercises to practice during the day (see Chapter 9 and page 254 for ideas). On your daily planner (pages 236-237), write down when you'll do them.

Plan to do relaxation exercises for 20 minutes, twice a day — first thing in the morning and then right before you prepare your evening meal. You may also want to add more relaxation time to your planner on days when your symptoms flare.

Spend your time wisely

Moderation and pacing are helpful techniques for managing your time — and in turn, managing fibromyalgia. That's because doing too much all at once, even if you're having a good day, may ultimately make your symptoms worse.

With these and other time-management skills, you can plan your day by balancing your activities and using your energy wisely. Time management can also help you keep stress from spiraling out of control.

Start by setting realistic goals around how you'll manage your time. Work with others — such as your co-workers, supervisor, friends and family — to set realistic expectations and deadlines. Making a priority list is another way to manage your time effectively. Prepare a list of tasks and rank them in order of priority. This can help you as you move through your day. Grouping similar tasks together can also help.

When you plan your day, think about the things that you need to do, the things that you want to do and the things you can do to take care of yourself. From there, balance all of those activities in a way that's realistic for you.

Start by looking at how you're spending your time now. On the next page, write down all of your current activities in a typical day in the left column. With this list, you'll start to see if you're making time for a variety of activities. Sure, work, exercise and

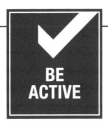

BE ACTIVE

MY CURRENT ACTIVITIES

MY ACTIVITY GOALS

responsibilities such as driving kids to school or activities and doing the laundry may be on your "current activities" list, but what about rest and relaxation? Do they make the list, as well?

Once you see how you typically spend your day, use the right column to set activity goals that can help you bring more variety into your day. This can help you balance your time and energy more effectively.

While you want to make sure to include "must-do" activities in your day, it's also important to do at least one fun activity a day. It's not selfish to do this — making time for rest, relaxation and enjoyment is critical to taking care of yourself.

Finally, do what you can to protect your time. For example, if you have an especially important or difficult project to work on, block out time to work on it without interruption. If you need a refresher, refer to the time-management tips in Chapter 14 to make the most of your time and your energy.

Plan it: Choose time-management strategies you would like to try and write them on your daily planner (pages 236-237).

Moderation, moderation, moderation

Moderation is key to helping you balance your activity level. It's also part of time management. By moderating activities in

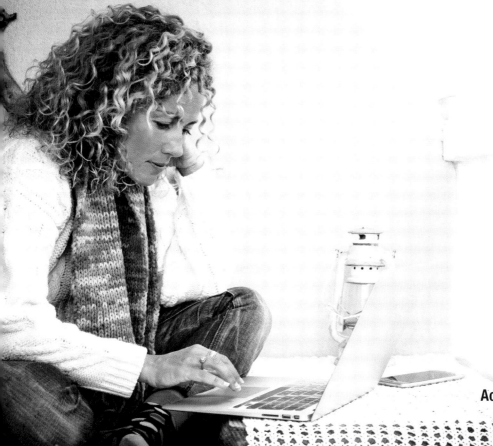

your life, you'll have enough energy when you need it, whether you're at work, relaxing, socializing or taking care of any task.

Plan it: Turn back to Chapter 14 for ideas on how you can moderate your activities. Find two that you would like to try and add them to your daily planner (pages 236-237).

Wind down, sleep well

You've set a regular time to wake up and a regular time to go to bed each day. Now it's time to think about how you can wind down before bedtime to ensure that you get good-quality rest. On page 178, you learned about steps you can take to get good sleep. Revisit these suggestions and choose a couple to try. Some of the relaxation exercises in Chapter 9 may also make your list.

Plan it: Once you've chosen the relaxation activities you would like to try, add them to your daily planner (pages 236-237).

Nurture your well-being

Each day, do one thing to improve your physical, emotional or spiritual well-being. This could mean spending time in prayer, practicing yoga or tai chi, visiting with someone you care about, taking time to laugh, or focusing on the present moment.

Plan it: Whatever you choose to do to improve your well-being, write it on your daily planner.

DIFFICULT DAYS

Bad days are bound to happen here and there. A bad day may mean you're feeling more pain than usual. Or, your physical health may not be a factor at all. Holidays are difficult for some people, for example. Unexpected events may also throw your day off track. Whatever the reason, you can handle a bad day. Planning to manage bad days is the best place to start.

Think of bad days that you've had recently. What made them bad? Extra stress, overdoing it and not getting enough physical activity can all lead to a bad day.

From there, use this information to help you identify warning signs. Can you think of things that signal that a bad day is coming? A headache or additional fatigue are both examples.

When you're having a bad day, stay connected. Don't isolate yourself from others. Stay on your usual schedule. Try to find distractions or diversions, and don't forget your relaxation techniques — spending more time using them can be helpful. Don't self-medicate, and above all, stay positive. Think back to past successes you've had in getting through a bad day — what you did then can help you now.

Use the checklist on page 233 the next time you're facing a difficult day. Fill it out, make a copy and post it where you can see it — perhaps by your phone — so it's nearby the next time you're facing a difficult day.

DIFFICULT DAYS

MY PLAN FOR DEALING WITH DIFFICULT DAYS

1. I will wake up and get out of bed on time.

2. I will do my morning stretches.

3. I will practice relaxation for 20 minutes. For example, I'll breathe. I'll use slow, regular-paced breathing. It calms me, and it helps me get rid of tension and pain.

4. I will say out loud, "This will pass," as often as I need to say it.

5. I will not change my current medications. I won't increase or decrease my dosages.

6. I won't drink alcohol or use other drugs.

7. I will exercise.

8. I will stay connected with people. Who in my social support network can I call if I'm having a difficult day?

   Name   Phone #

   Name   Phone #

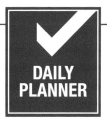

DAILY PLANNER

Use this example as a guide to create a daily planner of your own using the worksheet starting on page 236.

1. I will aim to get up at <u>6:30</u> a.m. each day.

2. I will do some gentle stretches after I get up, at <u>6:45</u> a.m. each day.

3. I will try to practice relaxation techniques for 20 minutes at <u>7</u> a.m. and <u>5:30</u> p.m.

4. I will try to walk or do one of the following physical activities for <u>10</u> minutes, <u>7</u> days a week:
- I will start walking for 10 minutes a day and increase my walking by two minutes every two weeks until I reach my goal of 30 minutes a day.

5. I will try these time-management methods:
- I will make a to-do list.
- I will set a timer so I can stay on track during the day.

6. I will try these stress-management methods:
- Relaxation exercises twice a day, 20 minutes each time, at 7 a.m. (first thing in the morning) and 5:30 p.m. (right before I prepare my evening meal).
- I will connect with friends because I know that social support is the biggest buffer against stress. I will connect with friends by taking a walk with a co-worker in the afternoon and calling a friend at night.

7. To keep me from doing too much or too little, I will change my activities in the following ways:
- I will schedule activities on my daily planner and I will set an alarm to tell me when it's time to take a break and to review my plan for my next activity.

8. I will change my bedtime routine in the following ways to help me relax:
- I will turn off all my screens, including the TV, one hour before I go to bed.
- I will take a bath to help me relax.

9. I will aim to go to bed at _10_ p.m. each day.

10. To help me improve my physical, emotional or spiritual health, I will try at least one of the following ideas each day:

- Plan to do something fun each day.
- Connect with a friend or family member each day.
- Get outside every day, even for just a short time, to connect with nature and my faith.

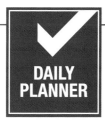

DAILY PLANNER

Use this worksheet to develop your daily plan.

1. I will aim to get up at _____ a.m. each day.

2. I will do some gentle stretches after I get up, at _____ a.m. each day. (Find stretching exercises starting on page 242.)

3. I will try to practice relaxation techniques for 20 minutes at _____ a.m. (first thing in the morning) and _____ p.m. (right before you prepare your evening meal).

4. I will try to walk or do one of the following physical activities for _____ minutes, _____ days a week: (See Chapter 13 if you need physical activity ideas.)

5. I will try these time-management methods: (Get ideas in Chapter 14.)

6. I will try these stress-management methods: (Get ideas in Chapter 15.)

7. To keep me from doing too much or too little, I will change my activities in the following ways: (Get ideas in Chapter 14.)

8. I will change my bedtime routine in the following ways to help me relax: (Revisit tips for a good night's sleep starting on page 178.)

9. I will aim to go to bed at _____ p.m. each day.

10. To help me improve my physical, emotional or spiritual health, I will try at least one of the following ideas each day:

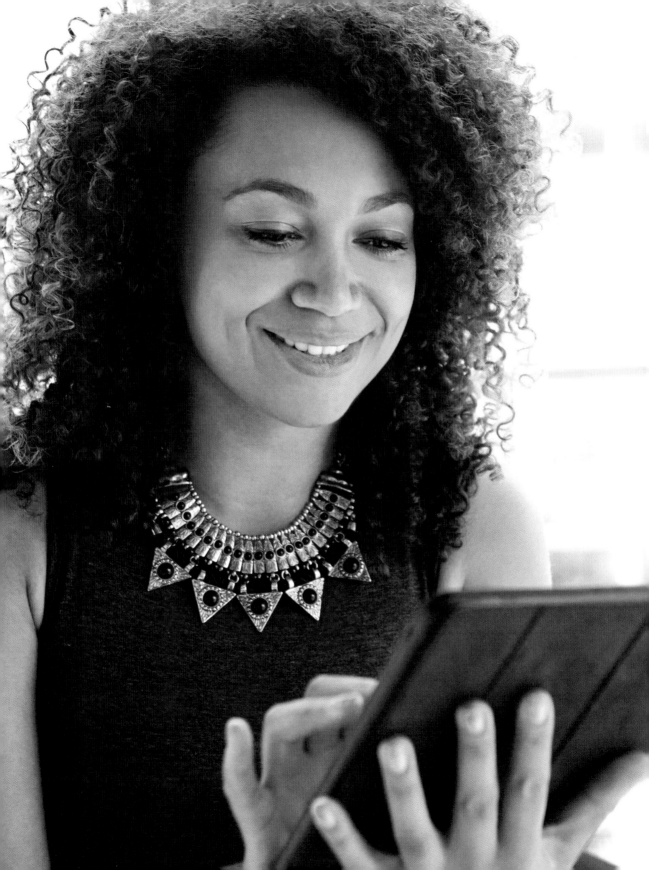

Additional resources

Find additional resources on fibromyalgia in this chapter, as well as worksheets to help you set your goals, stretching exercises, balance exercises and relaxation exercises.

This chapter offers tools to help you put your daily fibromyalgia plan into action.

SETTING GOALS

In Chapter 11, you learned about setting goals. As a reminder, when you set your goals, use the SMART acronym.

When you set a goal, make sure it's:

Specific State exactly what you want to achieve, when you want to achieve it and how you will do it.

Measurable Focus on clear outcomes you can measure. Plan to track your progress.

Attainable Make sure that you have the time and resources to devote to your goal.

Relevant Set goals that are meaningful and important to you and that fit your stage and style of life.

Time-limited Set a deadline for yourself.

On the next page, find an example of a SMART goal. Then use the worksheet on page 241 to set your own goals.

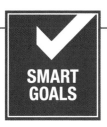

SMART GOALS

Let's say your goal is to start exercising. This alone, as a goal, is too vague. Here are ways you can make this goal SMART. Use this example to create a SMART goal of your own using the worksheet on the next page.

SPECIFIC
I will walk for 10 minutes after supper in the evening with my husband.

MEASURABLE
I will start with 10 minutes of walking and add two minutes every two weeks until I reach my goal of walking 30 minutes a day.

ATTAINABLE
I believe I can begin at 10 minutes. If it's too hard, I will cut back and start at 8 minutes a day instead.

RELEVANT
If I start walking, I will feel better and steadier on my feet. My ultimate goal is to walk to the grocery store near my house.

TIME-LIMITED
A daily walk, starting at 10 minutes a day and increasing by two minutes every two weeks, will help me reach my goal of walking 30 minutes a day, seven days a week.

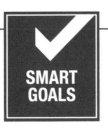

SMART GOALS

Use this worksheet to develop meaningful goals that can help you manage fibromyalgia symptoms. Copy this page and use it moving forward for any goal you want to set to yourself.

SPECIFIC

MEASURABLE

ATTAINABLE

RELEVANT

TIME-LIMITED

STRETCHING EXERCISES: HEAD AND NECK

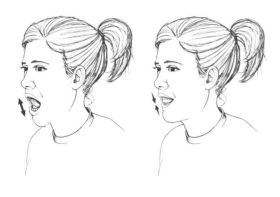

Jaw relaxation

1. Open and close your mouth.
2. Move your jaw from side to side.
3. Move your jaw from front to back.

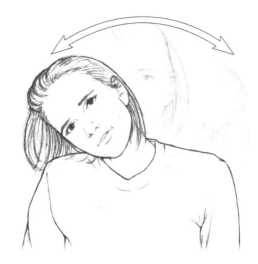

Neck stretch

1. Keep your face forward.
2. Tilt your head toward one shoulder.
3. Tilt your head toward the other shoulder.

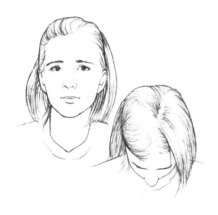

Chin tuck

1. Keep your body facing forward and your back straight.
2. Bring your chin toward your chest.
3. Return head to starting position.

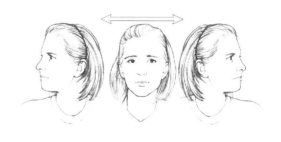

Head turn

1. Keep your body facing forward.
2. Turn your face to one side.
3. Turn your face to the other side.

STRETCHING EXERCISES: SHOULDERS

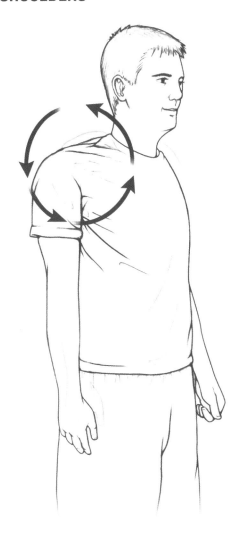

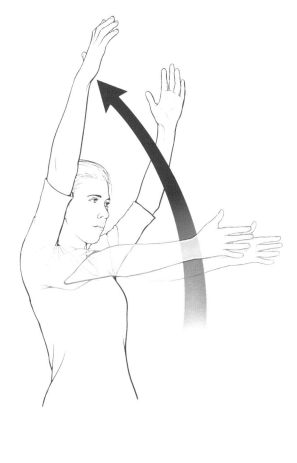

Arm extension to the front

1. Start with your arms at your sides.
2. Keep your thumbs pointed upward as you raise your arms straight out in front of you. Then raise your arms straight up. Stop when your arms are next to your ears.
3. Return your arms to your sides in the same way.

Shoulder roll

1. Keep your arms at your sides.
2. Roll your shoulders backward in a circular motion.
3. Roll your shoulders forward in a circular motion.

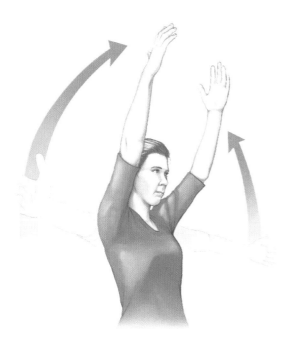

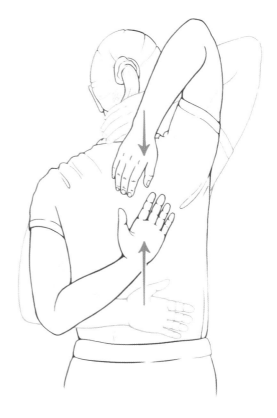

Arm extension to the side

1. Start with your arms at your sides.
2. Keep your thumbs pointed upward as you raise your arms straight out to your left and right sides. Then raise your arms straight up. Stop when your arms are close to your ears.
3. Return your arms to your sides in the same way.

Shoulder rotation stretch

1. Place the palm of your right hand on the back of your neck.
2. Place the back of your left hand in the curve of your back about waist high.
3. Try to touch your hands behind your back.
4. Switch hand positions. Place the palm of your left hand on the back of your neck. Place the back of your right hand in the curve of your back about waist high.
5. Try to touch your hands behind your back.

STRETCHING EXERCISES: TORSO

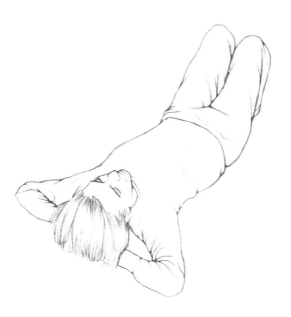

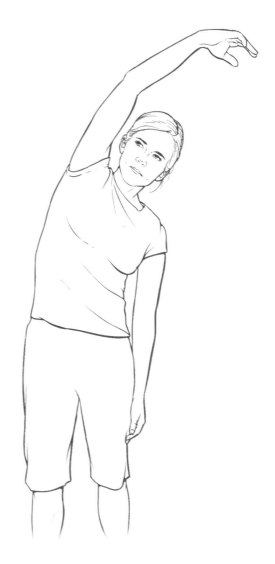

Upper chest stretch

1. Place the palms of your hands gently be-hind your head. Keep your hands on your head and do not push your head forward while you do this stretch.
2. Slowly breathe in as you pull your el-bows back as far as you can comfortably.
3. Slowly breathe out as you let your el-bows move forward and relax.

Side bend

1. Keep your body and head facing for-ward. Stand with your feet comfortably apart.
2. Lean to one side as you bring the oppo-site arm up over your head. Let your oth-er arm hang at your side.
3. Return to the starting position.
4. Repeat this stretch using your other side.

STRETCHING EXERCISES: ARMS AND WRISTS

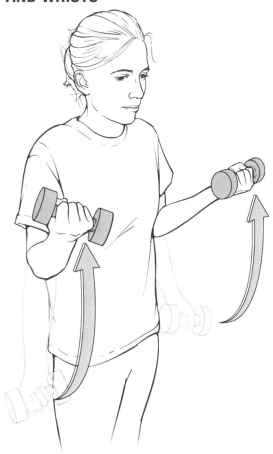

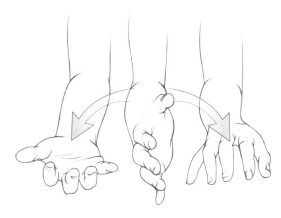

Wrist motion 1

1. Keep the upper part of your arm at the side of your body. Bend your elbow to form a right angle. Keep your elbow at your side.
2. Hold your hand out with your thumb up.
3. Turn your wrist so your palm faces up. Then turn your wrist so your palm faces down.

Bicep curls

1. Start with your arms at your side and your palms facing forward. Keep your upper arms next to your sides.
2. Moving only your lower arms, slowly raise your hands toward your shoulders. Stop before your hands reach your upper arms.
3. Keeping your upper arms next to your sides, slowly straighten your elbows and return your arms to the starting position.

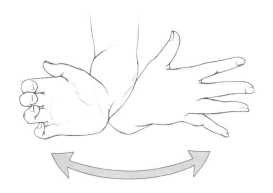

Wrist motion 2

1. Keep the upper part of your arm at the side of your body. Bend your elbow to

form a right angle. Keep your elbow at your side.

2. Hold your hand out with your thumb up.
3. Bend your wrist back and forth, toward and away from your body.
4. Repeat these steps for your other hand.

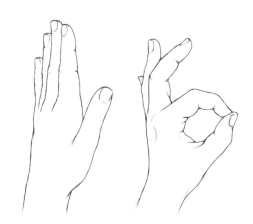

Thumb-to-finger opposition

1. Straighten your wrist and point your fingers and thumb upward.
2. Make an O shape by touching your index fingertip to your thumb.
3. Return to the starting position.
4. Repeat steps 2, 3 and 4 for each finger.
5. Repeat these steps for your other hand.

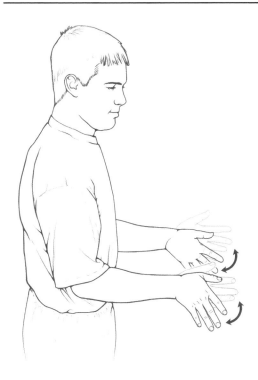

Karate chop

1. Keep the upper part of your arms at the side of your body.
2. Hold your hands out with your thumbs facing upward.
3. Bend your wrists to move your hands up and down. This movement is similar to a "karate chop."

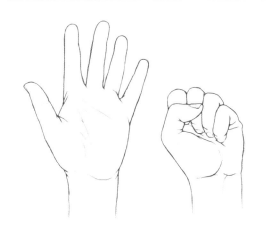

Make a fist

1. Curl your fingers in to make a fist.
2. Straighten your fingers.

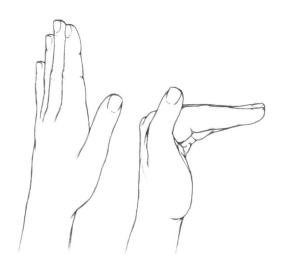 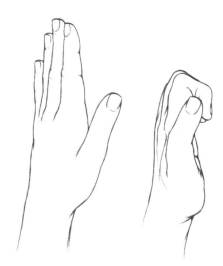

Tabletop (base-joint flexion)

1. Straighten your wrist and point your fingers and thumb up.
2. Bend the base joints (knuckles) of your fingers while keeping the end and middle joints and your wrist straight. This forms a "tabletop" with your hand.

Goal post (middle-joint and end-joint flexion)

1. Straighten your wrist and point your fingers and thumb upward.
2. Bend the end and middle joints of your fingers while keeping the base joints (knuckles) and your wrist straight.

STRETCHING EXERCISES: HIPS AND LEGS

Stand with your back straight to do these exercises. If you need help with balance, hold on to a counter or sturdy piece of furniture.

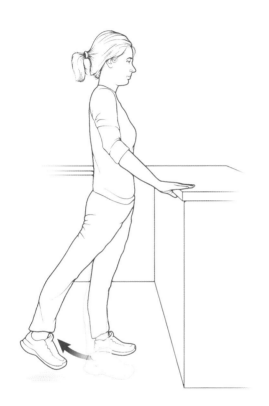

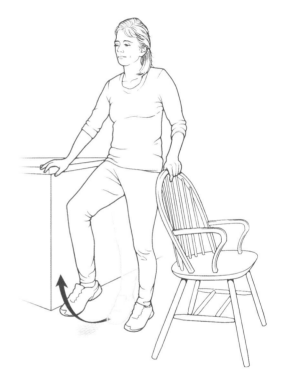

Hip extension

1. Move one leg straight back gently by lifting it and moving it backward. Keep your toes pointed forward and your leg straight as you do this.
2. Lower your leg.
3. Repeat these steps with your other leg.

Standing march

1. Spread your feet to be shoulder-width apart.
2. Bend one knee to lift the foot as high as you can.
3. Lower your foot.
4. Bend your other knee to lift your other foot.
5. Lower your foot.

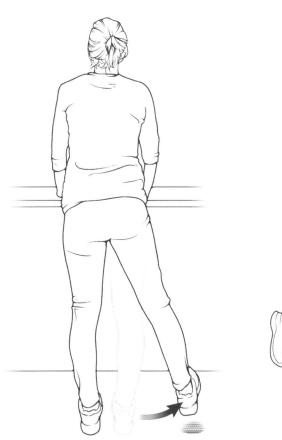

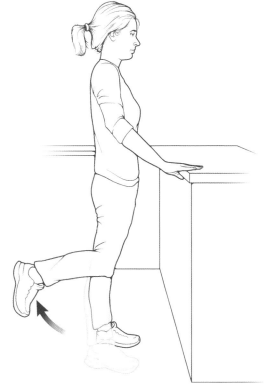

Hip abduction

1. Lift a leg and move it out to the side. Keep your toes pointed forward and your leg straight as you do this.
2. Lower your leg.
3. Repeat these steps with your other leg.

Knee flexion

1. Bend your knee to bring your foot toward your buttocks. Keep your upper leg still as you do this.
2. Lower your leg.
3. Repeat these steps with your other leg.

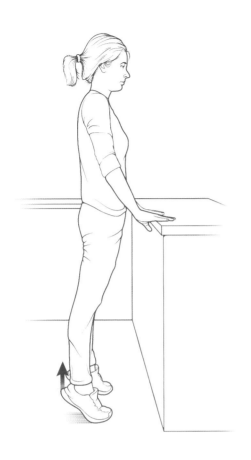

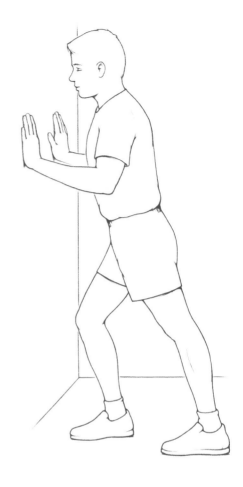

Heel lift

1. Keep your knees straight as you lift your heels as high as you can.
2. Slowly lower your heels to the floor.

Standing calf stretch

1. Stand with your hands pressing against a wall.
2. Move one leg back. Keep the knee straight and your foot flat on the floor.
3. Slightly bend your front leg. Lean on to that leg.
4. Hold the stretch for 15 to 30 seconds.
5. Return to starting position.
6. Repeat with your other leg.

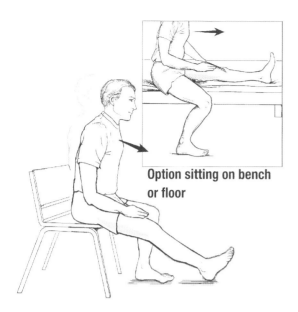

Option sitting on bench or floor

BALANCE

Stand to do these exercises. If you need help with balance, hold on to a counter or a sturdy piece of furniture.

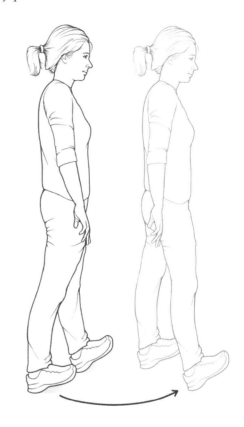

Sitting hamstring stretch

1. Sit on the front edge of a chair. Place one leg straight out in front of you with your heel on the floor and toes pointed upward. You may also sit on a firm surface, such as an exercise bench or the floor, to do this stretch.
2. Keep your back straight and slowly lean forward from your hips until you feel a stretch in the back of your straight leg.
3. Hold the stretch for 15 to 30 seconds.
4. Return to the starting position and relax.
5. Repeat these steps with your other leg.

1. Walk forward on your heels for 10 steps.

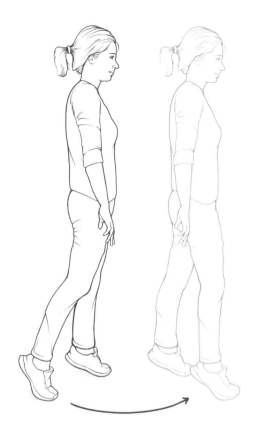

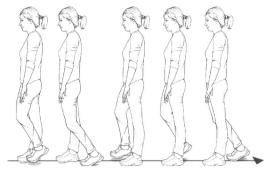

4. Walk backward in a straight line for 10 steps.

2. Walk forward on your toes for 10 steps.

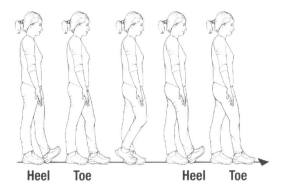

Heel   Toe   Heel   Toe

3. Walk forward for 20 steps in a straight line. Put your heel down first, then your toes. This is called walking heel to toe.

RELAXATION EXERCISES

On your daily planner (see page 236), schedule time for relaxation exercises to help calm your body and your mind. As a reminder, practice relaxation exercises for 20 minutes twice a day. Here are several to try.

Deep breathing

1. Lie on your back or sit comfortably with your feet flat on the floor.
2. Relax your shoulders as you breathe.
3. Breathe in slowly through your nose to a count of six. Allow your belly to expand. Your chest should move only slightly. Keep your shoulders relaxed.
4. Hold your breath for a count of one.
5. Breathe out slowly through your mouth to a count of six.

Repeat six to 10 times or as many times as you like.

Progressive muscle relaxation

1. Beginning with your face, squeeze the tiny muscles around your eyes, nose and mouth so that you form a tight grimace.
2. Hold the tension to the count of eight, exhale, and then allow your entire face to become loose and free.
3. Continue to move down your body, completely tensing your neck, then your jaw and then your shoulders. Hold each set of muscles for eight seconds and then release them.

4. Continue this exercise in your chest, arms, hands, fingers, belly, buttocks, legs, feet and toes until you've contracted and relaxed all of your muscle groups.

Short on time? Apply this technique to just a few targeted areas, such as your face and neck; arms, shoulders and belly; chest and buttocks; or legs and feet. Your larger muscle areas are contracted at once, rather than in smaller groups of muscles.

Guided imagery

1. Close your eyes, breathe deeply, and imagine yourself in a pleasant, peaceful place.
2. Use all of your senses. For example, watch the waves from the ocean wash over the shore of a sandy beach. Smell the salt water. Hear the sound of the waves crashing. Taste a long drink of cool water. Feel the sun's warmth on your skin.

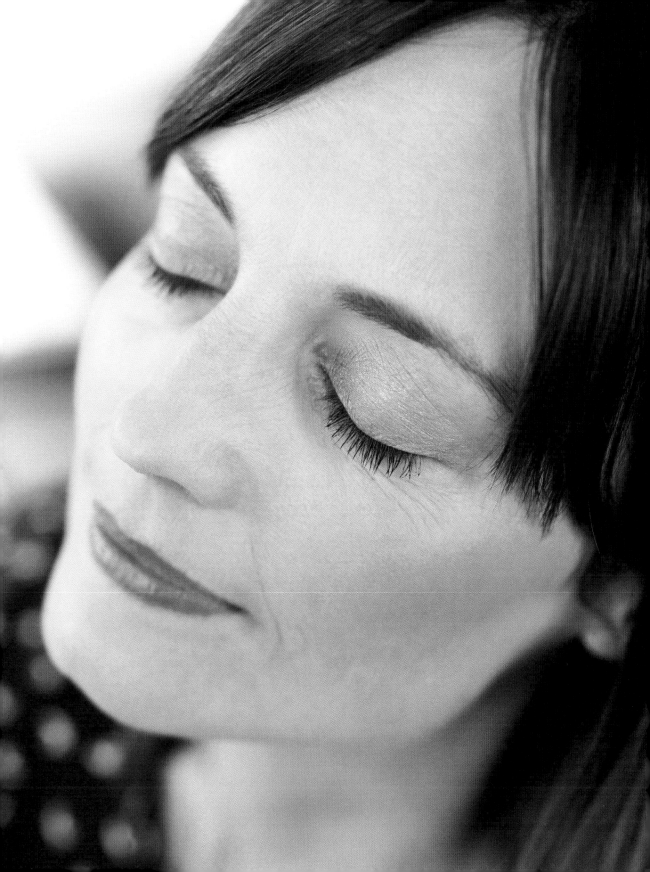

Other sources of information

AMERICAN ACADEMY OF PAIN MEDICINE

www.painmed.org/patientcenter
8735 W. Higgins Road, Suite 300
Chicago, IL 60631-2738
847-375-4731

AMERICAN CHRONIC PAIN ASSOCIATION

https://theacpa.org/condition/fibromyalgia
P.O. Box 850
Rocklin, CA 95677
800-533-3231

AMERICAN COLLEGE OF RHEUMATOLOGY

www.rheumatology.org/I-Am-A/Patient-Caregiver
2200 Lake Blvd. NE
Atlanta, GA 30319

AMERICAN PAIN SOCIETY

http://americanpainsociety.org
8735 W. Higgins Road, Suite 300
Chicago, IL 60631-2738
847-375-4715

ARTHRITIS FOUNDATION

www.arthritis.org/about-arthritis/types/fibromyalgia/
1355 W. Peachtree St. NE, Suite 600
Atlanta, GA 30309
800-283-7800

CENTERS FOR DISEASE CONTROL AND PREVENTION

www.cdc.gov/arthritis/basics/fibromyalgia.htm
1600 Clifton Road
Atlanta, GA 30329-4027
800-CDC-INFO (800-232-4636)

FIBROMYALGIA NETWORK

www.fmnetnews.com
P.O. Box 31750
Tucson, AZ 85751-1750
800-853-2929

INTERNATIONAL ASSOCIATION FOR THE STUDY OF PAIN

www.iasp-pain.org
1510 H St. NW, Suite 600
Washington, DC 20005-1020
202-856-7400

MAYO CLINIC

www.MayoClinic.org

MAYO CLINIC'S YOUTUBE CHANNEL

www.youtube.com/user/mayoclinic
Keyword search: fibromyalgia

NATIONAL CENTER FOR COMPLEMENTARY AND INTEGRATIVE HEALTH

https://nccih.nih.gov/health/pain/fibromyalgia. htm
9000 Rockville Pike
Bethesda, MD 20892
888-644-6226

NATIONAL FIBROMYALGIA & CHRONIC PAIN ASSOCIATION

www.fmcpaware.org
31 Federal Ave.
Logan, UT 84321
801-200-3627

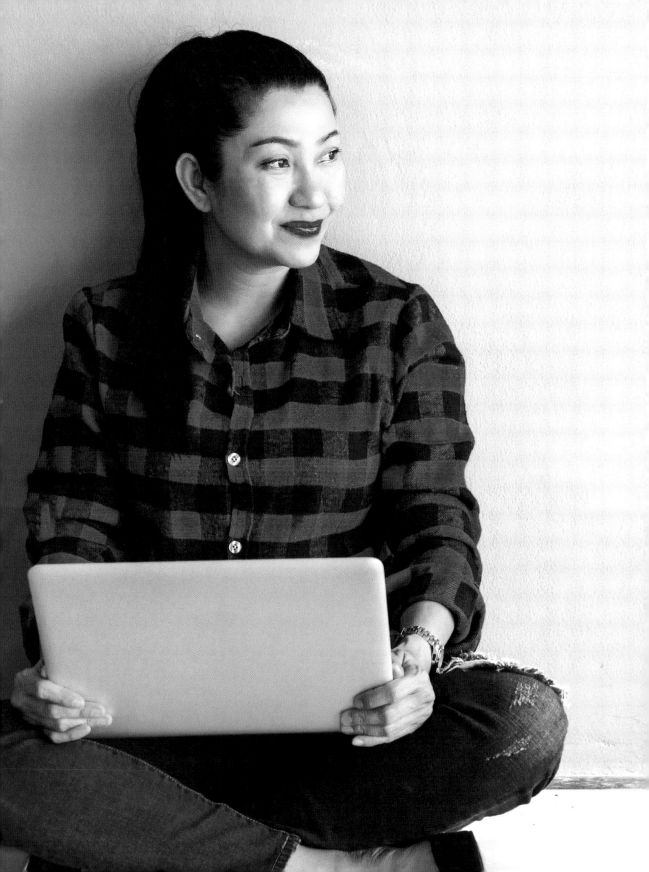

Glossary

A

acupuncture. The insertion of very thin needles through the skin at strategic points on the body. A key component of traditional Chinese medicine. Commonly used to treat pain by releasing the body's own pain-relieving chemicals (endorphins).

addiction. An illness in which a person seeks and consumes a substance, such as alcohol, tobacco or a drug, despite the fact that it causes harm.

aerobic exercise. Any movement that contracts large muscle groups, increases your heart rate and causes your lungs to work harder. Walking, swimming, biking, hiking, skiing, tennis and dancing are examples.

analgesic (an-ul-JEE-zik). A medication or agent that reduces pain.

anti-seizure medication. Used to treat fibromyalgia pain by affecting the body's pain pathways.

anxiety. How the body responds to stress. A common symptom of fibromyalgia.

B

balance exercises. Exercises that help maintain balance and prevent falls.

biofeedback. A relaxation technique that teaches the body to change its response to chronic pain and stress with the use of a special device.

brain fog. Thinking that feels faulty, memory problems or a short attention span. A common symptom of fibromyalgia. Also known as "fibro fog."

C

central sensitization. When communication between nerve sensors located throughout the body and your brain gets turned up (amplified). It makes ordinary sensations feel more intense. A light touch may hurt, a quiet noise may sound much louder than it usually does and lights may seem unbearably bright.

chronic pain. Pain that doesn't go away for three months or longer. It may or may not have an obvious cause.

cognitive behavioral therapy. Common type of talk therapy (psychotherapy). Helps you become aware of inaccurate or negative thinking so you can view challenging situations more clearly and respond to them in a more effective way.

D

deep breathing. A relaxation exercise in which you take deep, even-paced breaths using the muscle under your rib cage (diaphragm). Releases natural painkillers into the body and relaxes the muscles.

depression. A mood disorder that causes a persistent feeling of sadness and loss of interest. Common in people with fibromyalgia.

dual reuptake inhibitors/serotonin and norepinephrine reuptake inhibitors (SNRIs). One of two main types of antidepressants used to treat fibromyalgia. They affect chemicals in the brain that are responsible for helping to regulate and improve mood and reduce pain.

E

endorphins. Pain-relieving chemicals produced by the brain. They block pain signals and produce feelings of relaxation. Also called feel-good chemicals.

enkephalins (en-KEF-uh-lins). Naturally occurring molecules in the brain. Enkephalins attach to special receptors in your brain and spinal cord to stop pain messages. They also affect other functions within the brain and nervous system.

F

fibromyalgia. A chronic pain disorder characterized by widespread musculoskeletal pain accompanied by fatigue as well as sleep, memory and mood issues. Amplifies painful sensations by affecting the way the brain processes pain signals.

G

guided imagery. A relaxation exercise that enlists the power of the imagination to take you to places you find relaxing. Used to help people feel more at ease and feel less pain.

H

hyperalgesia. Abnormally increased pain sensation.

hydrotherapy. The use of warm or hot water to relax muscles and ease tension. Also called balneotherapy.

I

inflammation. The protective response of body tissues to irritation or injury. May be acute or chronic. Signs and symptoms are redness, heat, swelling and pain, often accompanied by loss of function.

integrative medicine. The practice of using conventional medicine along with complementary treatments that have been shown to help manage or treat a condition.

interdisciplinary pain management programs. Programs that bring together several therapies and experts in an integrated and targeted fashion. They focus on helping improve daily functioning and quality of life.

interstitial cystitis. A condition that causes pain and pressure in the bladder, frequent urination, and pelvic pain. Common in people with fibromyalgia.

irritable bowel syndrome. A disorder that causes chronic belly pain and a change in bowel habits. As many as half of people with fibromyalgia also have irritable bowel syndrome.

M

massage therapy. Manipulation of the soft tissues of your body — muscle, connective tissue, tendons, ligaments and skin — using varying degrees of pressure and movement. A type of integrative medicine used to treat pain.

meditation. A relaxation exercise that involves calmly focusing on the present moment to help quiet the mind and relax the muscles.

moderation. A time-management approach for conserving energy. It means not doing too much on good days and not doing too little on bad days. Moderation and pacing are used together to balance energy.

moving meditation. Relaxation exercises that combine physical activity with meditation. Yoga, tai chi, qi gong and Pilates are examples.

muscle relaxers. A type of medication used to treat mild to moderate fibromyalgia symptoms. Used to help promote sleep. Thought to help with fibromyalgia symptoms in a way that's similar to antidepressants.

N

neuroplasticity. Changes in the brain that happen when you learn new things, experience changes or adapt to the world around you.

nodules. Hardened areas of muscle that are painful to the touch.

O

occupational therapist. A skilled professional who helps people return to ordinary tasks around home and at work by way of lifestyle adaptations and occasionally with the aid of assistive devices.

off-label drugs. Drugs that are not approved by the Food and Drug Administration for treatment of fibromyalgia but are sometimes prescribed to help relieve symptoms.

opioids. A broad group of pain-relieving drugs that interact with opioid receptors in the body's cells. Made from the poppy plant or in a laboratory.

P

pacing. A time-management approach for conserving energy. Involves alternating activities that require energy with periods of rest. Pacing and moderation are used together to balance energy.

peripheral nerves. Nerves that run from your spinal cord to all other parts of your body. They transmit messages from the spinal cord and brain to and from other parts of your body and send sensory signals back to the spinal cord and brain. Damage to these nerves can lead to miscommunication about pain getting to the brain.

physical deconditioning. Being unable to move the body as well as usual when the muscles haven't been used.

physical dependence. The physical condition in which rapid discontinuation of a substance — such as alcohol, tobacco or a drug — causes a withdrawal reaction.

physical therapist. A trained professional who teaches exercises and other physical activities to aid in rehabilitation and maximize physical ability with less pain.

progressive muscle relaxation. A relaxation exercise in which body parts are tightened and then relaxed one at a time, in sequence.

R

rheumatism. Pain, discomfort, soreness and stiffness in the joints and muscles that can affect how easily you move.

rheumatologist. A doctor who focuses on arthritis and other similar conditions. A rheumatologist diagnoses fibromyalgia after ruling out other problems first.

S

selective serotonin reuptake inhibitors (SSRIs). Medications used to relieve depression. Thought to work by increasing the availability of a brain chemical (serotonin) that helps to regulate mood. Sometimes used to treat fibromyalgia.

serotonin (ser-o-TOE-nin). A brain chemical (neurotransmitter) that helps to regulate mood. A lack of it may lead to depression.

SMART. A goal-setting strategy. Stands for Specific, Measurable, Attainable, Relevant and Time-limited.

strength training. Any exercise that builds muscles. May involve resistance against body weight or activities that involve the use of hand-held weights, machine weights, or exercise bands. Yoga is another example.

stress. A natural reaction to something threatening. Also a natural reaction to welcomed events in life. Causes the heart to race and blood pressure to rise.

stretches. Exercises that increase range of motion. Used to prevent injury and help relieve stiffness.

T

temporomandibular joint (TMJ) dysfunction. Pain in the joint and muscles around the jaw with no sign of injury.

tender points. Areas of the body that hurt or are sensitive to the touch when pressure is applied. Someone with fibromyalgia may have tender points, but people who have tender points may not have fibromyalgia.

thalamus. A part of the brain that relays impulses from the sensory nerves. Sensory nerves allow people to feel pain.

the Americans with Disabilities Act. A federal civil rights law that prevents job discrimination for people with certain disabilities. Protects people in areas such as hiring, firing, advancement, compensation and job training. Specific medical conditions, such as fibromyalgia, aren't listed under the Americans with Disabilities Act.

the Family Medical Leave Act. A federal law that allows employees with qualifying family or medical reasons to take unpaid leave for up to 12 weeks without losing their job.

tolerance. When your body gets used to the dose of medication you're taking, causing you to increase the dose of medication over and over again to achieve the same level of pain relief.

tricyclic antidepressants. A group of drugs used to relieve symptoms of depression that may also help relieve pain. One of two main types of antidepressants used to treat fibromyalgia.

trigger points. Areas of the body that, when touched, cause pain in other parts of the body.

W

widespread pain. Pain throughout the body, near pathways that lead to the brain. A common symptom of fibromyalgia.

withdrawal. The physical or psychological state experienced when certain substances or medications are discontinued rapidly.

Index

treatment

    changing approach to, 95–96

    cognitive behavioral therapy, 95–101

    integrative medicine, 103–111

    interdisciplinary pain management
        programs, 113–119

    medications, 81–93

trigger points, 22

triggers, 41, 47, 131, 187, 211

W

weakness, 48, 64

widespread pain, 58

work issues, 69, 217–222

Y

yoga, 107, 108, 144

IMAGE CREDITS

The individuals pictured are models, and the photos are used for illustrative purposes only. There is no correlation between the individuals portrayed and the subjects being discussed.

All photographs and illustrations are copyright of MFMER, except for the following:

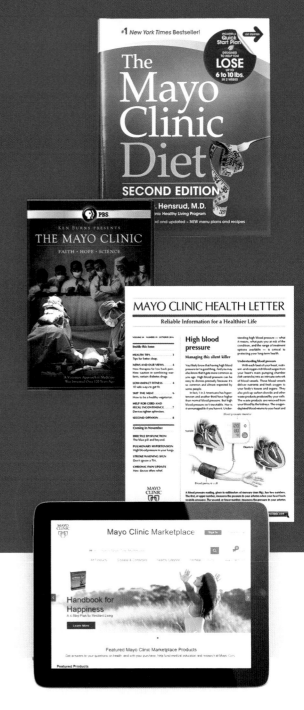

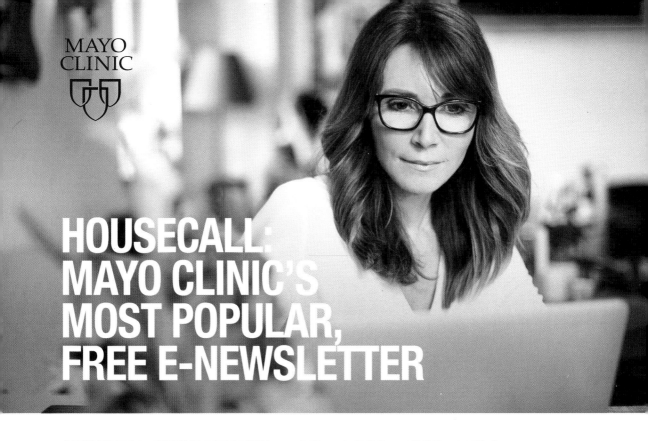

HOUSECALL: MAYO CLINIC'S MOST POPULAR, FREE E-NEWSLETTER

GET THE LATEST HEALTH & WELLNESS INFORMATION FROM MAYO CLINIC DELIVERED DIRECTLY TO YOUR EMAIL.

I depend on Mayo Clinic Housecall more than any other medical info that shows up on my computer.

Excellent newsletter. I always find something interesting to read and learn something new.

I love Housecall. It is one of the most useful, trusted and beneficial things that comes from the internet.

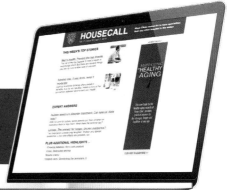

SIGN UP TODAY AT
MayoClinic.com/housecall/register

MAYO CLINIC | mayoclinic.org